Finally,
Dreams Coming True

Jacqueline Speciner
Phyllis Godwin

Acknowledgments

We would like to thank Crosby King for his help in editing parts of this book. We appreciate his time, effort, and hard work.

We would also like to express our appreciation to author boice–Terrel Allen for his professional publishing advice. His expertise was extremely helpful.

Authors' Note

The names of many of the people in this memoir have been changed. This has been done to protect the privacy of certain individuals.

Finally,
Dreams Coming
True

I

One January day in 1958, someone made a mistake that would permanently alter my life. It was a costly mistake for both of us. She paid for it with her job, but I paid a much higher price.

The mistake was caused by a misunderstanding. Some misunderstandings can be resolved with a simple phone call and a few quick words of explanation and apology. Others can be of such monumental proportions that the consequences can be life changing. It all began with a mistake and a misunderstanding – and the few short minutes it took for them to occur created many challenges in my life.

II

My parents were quite young when I was born. My 17 year old mother, practically a child herself, gave birth to me on January 11, 1958 in Baltimore, Maryland. I, Jacqueline Anne Leimbach, entered this world two months prematurely, weighing only two pounds. Due to my early arrival and low birth weight, I was immediately placed in an incubator. It was imperative that I stay there to sustain my tiny body outside of my mother's womb.

Three days after I was born, another patient in the hospital was looking for the nursery. My mother politely offered to show her the way. As they were walking down the hallway, a nurses' aide spotted my mother, and mistakenly assumed that she wanted to hold me. Unfortunately, the aide removed me from the incubator. Immediately, they both realized the seriousness of her actions. The short amount of time that I was out, deprived of the oxygen that my brain so desperately needed, resulted in my having cerebral palsy. And so began a life full of extremes for me – of joyful times and horrific times, of caregivers and abusers, of satisfaction and frustration.

III

Since I was her first child, my mother didn't know exactly what to expect in the way of my development. She was aware, however, that I was not progressing like other babies she had seen. She first became concerned when she noticed that I wasn't able to hold my head up properly, and her concern turned to anxiety when I was old enough to sit up alone but couldn't. She began taking me to one doctor after another searching for answers, not realizing that my time out of the incubator was the cause of my difficulties.

It took two full years for my mother to finally find the answer. Until then, she was brushed off by doctors who would tell her: You worry too much! You are a new mother, and you are overanxious. All babies are different. You are watching her too closely! There's nothing wrong with her. She's just taking her time! But, my mother refused to accept their explanations, and continued her quest for the truth.

Finally, when I was two years old, Dr. Jenkins *did* come up with the right answer. His diagnosis was that I had cerebral palsy, and it was due to oxygen deprivation to my brain. Naturally, my parents were stunned and took his pronouncement terribly hard. Additionally, my mother had feelings of guilt to deal with, since she felt responsible for my being out of the incubator. Both of my parents knew in their hearts that something was wrong, but they were not expecting such devastating news - news that would affect their firstborn child for the rest of her life.

Dr. Jenkins may have made the correct diagnosis of my problem but he definitely made the wrong suggestion for how my parents should handle me. He strongly recommended that they place me in an institution. He had a tremendously negative outlook and extremely poor attitude for a doctor. He had no encouraging words to say about my possible prospects for a productive life. In his practice, he had many patients with cerebral palsy – and the first thing he told all of their families was to put them away. They'll never be contributing citizens to society! They'll never make a positive impact in their communities! They are not worth the trouble of caring for them. Just put them away!

To this day, I am so grateful that my parents chose not to follow his advice. Although it has been a long and sometimes arduous journey for me, I have also experienced joy and many accomplishments in my life. And, I have had the satisfying opportunity to prove Dr. Jenkins to be very wrong!

IV

Flashbulbs were going off! There was primping and posing for photographs! There were celebrities, and I was even traveling! All of this excitement surrounded a thrilling part of my childhood – and I adored every moment of it! At the tender age of three, I became the poster child for United Cerebral Palsy! I felt proud and greatly honored to be chosen for that distinction. My tenure as poster child lasted two glorious years, and during that time I traveled all over Maryland promoting United Cerebral Palsy. I was privileged to meet celebrities and sports figures, including Baltimore Colts Hall of Famer, Gino Marchetti. There was much celebration and applause at the ceremony on Cold Spring Lane when I was the lucky one who had the honor of breaking the ground for the agency's new facility! For a small child with a physical challenge, the attention I received was exhilarating!

Unfortunately, soon after this happy period of my life, a major disappointment followed. My father was on the road almost constantly, traveling for his job. His long absences from home put a tremendous strain on my mother. While he was gone, she had the full responsibility of caring for me on her own, and by that time, another daughter Janice, as well. It was a hardship for her, and it took its toll. My parents separated when I was five years old, and divorced soon after. This was heartbreaking for me because I loved my father very much, and I knew for a fact that he adored me.

V

Shortly after the divorce, my mother remarried. Marrying someone who has a child with a physical challenge is a huge, long-term commitment. Unfortunately, not everyone considers the ramifications that this entails. Sadly, my mother's new husband Earl was not prepared for the drastic changes I would make in his life. He made it clear immediately that I was nothing but an enormous inconvenience to him. He resented the care that I needed and thought I was in the way all the time. And unfortunately, his actions proved time and time again, exactly how he felt.

My stepfather had very little patience with me, and he would get angry about things that I couldn't help. My mother had me potty trained at three years old, and by the time I was five, I could communicate very well to her when I needed to use the bathroom. However, like any other child, I had occasional accidents. Sometimes, I would wet myself while laughing with my sister and this would infuriate Earl.

Later on, a surgical mistake affected the muscle elasticity of my intestines. This caused me to lose control of my bowels which upset Earl even more. Since this was a new problem for me, my mother was concerned and called the doctor. Instead of admitting that a surgical error was at fault, his response was that "Jacquie must be getting retarded." That one insensitive statement broke my heart. My sisters and friends began teasing me about being retarded – something they had never done before – and it added more fuel to the fire for my stepfather. He became even less tolerant of me and my needs.

Sadly, my mother and stepfather saw me differently than their other children. If their attitude toward me had been more positive, my insecurities might not be so severe today. Although my mother didn't consider me an inconvenience to herself, she never wanted anyone else to have to take care of me. She thought I was a burden and a bother to other people. If someone did help me, my mother expected me to appreciate whatever they did, even if I didn't like it. She drummed this into my head over and over again. To this day, she still thinks I should be grateful for anything and everything that comes my way. I can't agree with her viewpoint though. Just because I live with physical challenges, doesn't mean I shouldn't have input concerning what happens to me. I am a person – first and foremost – and I have opinions and preferences. And I have the right to express them just like everyone else!

VI

Most children look forward to starting school, and I was no exception. In fact, I wanted to be there more than anywhere else. I started kindergarten in a school for children with physical challenges, and graduated after I completed the 12th level when I was 22 years old. I loved my school because it was full of special people who truly cared for me. It was also an escape from the misery I endured at home.

My school years were wonderful ones for me. I got along well with the other students, and enjoyed being with them every day. My two best subjects, science and music, excited me and I particularly loved being in the school choir. Sometimes, my singing at home and on the school bus made people wish I had an "off" button. But despite everyone's negative opinion of my vocal talent, my parents knew that being in the choir was good for me. I was still proud of my performances, and delighted that my family came to see me.

School field trips were especially fun because my grandmother would go along, too. She was much more involved with me at school than my parents. My favorite trips were to plays, musicals, and art museums because they involved my senses of sight and hearing. It made me feel more like everyone else if I didn't have to read.

Reading was laborious for me. I was taught the sounds one at a time, but it was grueling work. Although I couldn't help myself, I often got into trouble for not staying focused. I was easily distracted by my surroundings, and no matter how hard I tried to look straight at the teacher, that didn't always work. I became impatient, and I didn't want to take the time to learn to read. Even though I was frustrated, I listened carefully to everything, and slowly began to memorize the words of stories.

Eventually, it seemed like I was reading when I was actually just reciting the words by heart.

School was terribly difficult because of my lack of concentration, but I did my best and worked hard. It often took me a long time to complete a task. I would always try to finish my class work before the bell rang at the end of the day. If I did, I felt a great sense of accomplishment. But if I didn't, that was okay, too. Incomplete class work became homework, and I *loved* doing homework! My sisters would tease me about that all the time. If someone would sit down and help me, I wanted to get right to it the minute I came in the door. I know that's unusual, but that's how I was!

Lots of children dread when their parents have conferences with their teachers or go to PTA meetings. But I actually loved when those meetings were scheduled! I knew the teachers would say positive things, and it was an opportunity for my parents to hear good news about me. That made me ecstatic!

Memories of school and my teachers are such pleasant ones! I was treated well and I relished the one on one attention that I received there. My teachers Miss Dardell, Miss Prector, and Miss Beck were extremely kind. I also had a dedicated physical therapist who really had her work cut out for her. She did my stretching exercises with me in school, but unfortunately, my mother was not continuing my therapy at home. This caused my joints to stiffen up, making it more difficult for my therapist to help me. Had my mother followed up consistently with my exercises, maybe it would have slowed down my loss of mobility.

My mother was only bathing me once a week, so it was not unusual for me to come to school soiled with feces. At first, the staff would write notes to my family complaining about it, but it didn't take them long to realize that their messages were causing trouble for me at home. Once they were aware of that, they immediately stopped sending the notes. Instead, they started handling the situation themselves. One staff member in particular took it upon herself to clean me up whenever I arrived dirty. She was the physical therapy aide, and her name was Livvie Maddox. I called her my "soul mother" and I will never forget her. She will always have a special place in my heart. Because of all these nurturing individuals, school was a safe, secure environment, and therefore became a refuge for me.

Although my mother neglected many of my needs, I remember a time when she participated in something very important to me. From the age of seven until I was nine years old, I belonged to a Brownie Girl Scout troop. It was especially enjoyable for me because my mother helped the leader. I was thrilled beyond belief that she was involved in this activity with me. Getting out of my house and socializing with other girls was also something I looked forward to each week. It was fun and rewarding to learn new skills, and I was so proud each time I successfully completed a project. With each accomplishment, I hoped my mother was noticing my success. I felt such satisfaction when I won awards. All of this helped boost my self-esteem which I so desperately needed.

VII

Some of my happiest memories are of times spent with my paternal grandmother. She often invited me to spend the weekend with her, and I was grateful for the opportunity to get away from home for a couple of days. Weekends at my grandmother's house were a special treat for me because she loved me unconditionally, and enjoyed spoiling me. She'd give me just about anything I wanted, and cooked all of my favorite foods. She even took the time to do my physical therapy. It was a very different atmosphere from my house. I was so happy there that I never wanted to leave, and unfortunately, every visit ended the same way.

On my last day there, I would undergo a drastic mood change. I would become miserable and angry. I'd cry and throw temper tantrums. My family misunderstood my reactions, and thought I was behaving childishly. I appeared unappreciative, but that couldn't have been farther from the truth. I just did not want to go home, and the fact that I had no choice in the matter frustrated me in a way that no one understood. But how could they? How could they understand or know how I felt? How could they know what it was like to have all of their decisions made for them? They could make their own choices every day. I didn't have that luxury. Choices were always being made *for* me.

VIII

I did, however, choose to have boyfriends. People are often surprised to learn that someone with a physical challenge even *has* a boyfriend. I am a woman, and I have all of the same feelings and physical needs as every other woman. I'm not sure why that is such a difficult notion for people to grasp. I need love, affection, and yes – even sex, regardless of my body's condition. Sex is not a dirty word. It is not some kind of voodoo magic. The desire for sex is just as healthy for me as it is for any able-bodied person.

I met my first boyfriend Carlos when I was 16 years old. We were in the Catoctin Mountains at Camp Greentop, a camp for people with challenging physical conditions. Carlos was physically fit, and that is another concept that people find hard to imagine. Why would a perfectly able-bodied young man want to go out with a girl in a wheelchair? Because thankfully, Carlos saw beyond the wheelchair to the girl, and he liked what he saw.

Carlos and I dated for three years, but it was a difficult courtship. Although Carlos did not discriminate against me because of my challenges, unfortunately my parents were not as open-minded about him. He was Puerto Rican and that was a big issue with them. He was never allowed to come into our house, and always had to meet me outside. It was hurtful to Carlos, but it did not discourage him. He knew the situation in my home was less than ideal, so he took me out shopping and to the movies as often as possible. He was extremely protective of me, too. Our dating was also very regimented due to the strict curfew imposed by my parents. If we were ever late, we were subjected to lengthy questioning.

Despite all of the obstacles, Carlos continued to see me until he found out that my mother had arranged for me to have a hysterectomy when I was 18 years old. He was angry with her for her actions, but even angrier with me for allowing it to happen. He thought I should have resisted my mother's decision. He didn't understand that, at that time, it never would have occurred to me to question her, or refuse to obey. I was still living in her house, and I didn't think I had a choice in the matter. Carlos was a good and loyal friend for three years, and I believe that eventually he could have been even more than that. However, he couldn't get over what I had let my mother do to me, and so he ended our relationship.

IX

In my mother's eyes, I was never a woman. That could explain how arranging for me to have a hysterectomy at 18 years old didn't seem the least bit inappropriate to her. Her denial of my womanhood probably also contributed to the fact that she never told me about my menstrual cycle. She was uncomfortable – and still is today – talking about such private matters. I was at camp the first time I got my period, and had absolutely no knowledge of what was happening. When I saw the blood, I naturally assumed that I was bleeding to death. One of my camp counselors explained everything to me and bought me some sanitary supplies. She then reprimanded my mother for not preparing me for this major occurrence in my life.

After that, I was not allowed to go out on a date if I had my period. My mother thought that men should not see women in that condition since their bodies were cleaning themselves. Thankfully, I had a more insightful source of information at school, and later one of my teachers explained to me about living with the natural functions of my body.

My legs were together so tightly because of my cerebral palsy, that it was difficult for my mother to change my sanitary pads. This is the reason she wanted me to have the hysterectomy. Truthfully, at the time I wasn't really bothered by her decision. It wasn't until after I was married that I realized the importance of what I had given up.

This is a perfect example of why I feel that by 16 or 17 years old, children with challenging conditions should move out of their parents' home. It's an ideal age to start becoming more independent, and begin making decisions for themselves. If I had been on my own at the time, it's possible that I may have never had a hysterectomy.

And besides, although it's not a pleasant thought, parents are not immortal. Everyone should be realistic. It's best to prepare ahead of time, so that finding an alternative place to live does not turn into an emergency situation that must be accomplished overnight, possibly by strangers. Planning for the future makes for a much smoother transition into new surroundings.

Making time to do some research beforehand, gives you a chance to find a place where you feel comfortable. Your family should help you with this, so they can look out for your best interests. This is the most efficient way to handle the situation because if you wait too long, you may not have any say about where you end up living. If you are still at home with your parents when they pass away, you could be put somewhere that you don't like. On the other hand, while your parents are alive, they can see the home you have chosen, make sure you have everything you need, and that you are happy.

When you are considering an apartment, be aware that although you are told it is accessible, that may not be a completely accurate statement. Being accessible does not mean just being able to get through the front door. According to the Americans with Disabilities Act, all doorways must be 36 inches wide. In addition, the apartment should have roll in showers and raised countertops.

The location of the apartment is a critical consideration, and should play a major part in your final selection. If you are physically capable of using public transportation, make sure you are in an area where that is available. Is the apartment close to your school, shopping, your doctors, and banks? If you utilize a wheelchair, can you safely get to those places without having to cross busy or dangerous roads? Check on these details yourself, and don't take someone else's word for it.

I made that mistake once, and found myself stuck in an apartment that was totally inaccessible to everything I needed. David, a supervisor at United Cerebral Palsy, told me that it was in a good location, but I found out too late that was a lie. It was not even on a bus line which caused huge transportation headaches for my personal care attendants. One of my favorite attendants Noel, who had health problems of her own, would have to get a cab to my place during the week. This ended up costing her more than her salary. On weekends, her parents would have to bring her, and she would stay overnight at my apartment. At times, when no one could get there, I would spend three or four days home alone.

Also, in order to get to my bank, I had to risk my life crossing over a multi-lane highway. My personal care attendant and I did that once, but she said she would not take a chance like that again. From then on, she would have to lift me from my wheelchair into a cab and put the wheelchair back in my apartment before we rode to the bank. It was terribly inconvenient and difficult for her. Fortunately, the bank tellers understood my needs. They would come out to the cab, and conduct my financial business there. Although everyone was extremely accommodating, it was a cumbersome situation.

When I complained about the location to United Cerebral Palsy, David said the apartment manager told him that the complex was on a bus line. I later found out that was not true, and that the manager told David anyone living there would most definitely need a car. I ended up having to stay there for a year, feeling completely isolated. I was angry with David for lying to me, and that's when my faith in United Cerebral Palsy started a downhill slide. So, always be sure to thoroughly investigate the location of the apartment you are considering *in person*, if at all possible. Be absolutely certain that it is where you want, and need, to be.

When you are in the market for an apartment, I would strongly suggest that someone else go with you – a parent or another person you trust. Have that person take notes for you, and record the answers to all of your questions. This can help avoid confusion later on.

Request that all important information be put into whatever form is most helpful to you. If you need the lease to be written in large print, Braille, or even tape recorded, insist on it. It's your legal and constitutional right! It must be precise, and easy for you to comprehend.

Don't make a final decision based only on what you personally are told. After *your* meeting with the rental agent, send an able-bodied decoy there, and have her express interest in renting an apartment, too. Compare notes later, to see if she received the identical information and answers that you did. This will assist you in determining if the management is guilty of discrimination of any kind. Discrimination against people with physical challenges does exist, and unfortunately can lead to lies and intentional misrepresentation. I lost the best apartment I ever had after just three months, because I was misled regarding Section 8 eligibility. Make sure you completely understand *everything*!

X

Moving into your own place, gives you the opportunity to incorporate your personal interests into your life. It also allows you to make decisions about what you want to do and where you want to go. You can even choose not to go along on family vacations.

My mother and stepfather Earl had a vacation house in West Virginia. As much as I loved to go away, I really disliked those particular trips. Although it was supposed to be a family outing, I was never included in any of the family activities while we were there. Everyone would go about having their own fun, and I would just sit alone in the house. I was even left behind when they all went to the swimming pool.

These vacations were so boring to me that by the time I was in my early 20's, I started thinking of ways to get out of them. My family wasn't about to just let me stay home, so I had to come up with a plan. I was at such a point of frustration that I would do almost anything to avoid going.

One Friday, as I was leaving my day program, I made a spontaneous decision. I knew that when I got home, I'd be packed into the car and whisked away to another monotonous weekend in West Virginia. Instead of riding the bus home, I took it to my boyfriend Neil's house. We had met two years before, and I decided that I was staying there until Monday. I called my mother so she wouldn't worry, and although she was furious, she did not come to get me. And so, at 22 years old, I finally displayed a show of independence and made it clear to everyone that I had a mind of my own.

XI

Shortly after that, I decided to move out of my parents' house. I was going to live in an apartment with two other women and staff from United Cerebral Palsy. I was anxious for this next phase of my life to begin, but people were skeptical about my chances for success in a new environment - especially my parents. My family did not think this arrangement would last, and expected me to be back home in a week. They didn't believe that anyone else was capable of taking care of me.

Although I was enthusiastic about my new apartment, it was still a frightening step for me to take. Actually, I should call it a frightening *leap*. As I was about to leave home, I began to feel some separation anxiety and concern. Not knowing exactly who was going to take care of me was a huge worry. Like anyone else, I was afraid of the unknown. I took a deep breath though and got on the bus. Then I happily waved good-bye to my family. They were stunned that I was smiling instead of crying when I left. In fact, I think they were quite upset that I looked so cheerful as the bus pulled away! It was obvious that I was glad to be going.

This is not to say that I didn't have any sad moments after I moved, or that I was never homesick. To tell the truth, I did cry the first night I was gone because I already missed my mother, and wasn't sure when I'd see her again. I cried a few more times in the early days, but the sadness lessened as I adjusted to my new way of life.

Naturally, I was thrilled to be in my own apartment. After all, I was an adult, and it was time. I was soon to find out however, that like many situations in life, it had positive aspects but also drawbacks.

Sharing that first apartment with my roommates Rosalie and Odessa was wonderful. Although I was the youngest by about 20 years, we all got along remarkably well together. As time went by, the three of us became more than just residents in the same home. We became friends, and looked out for each other.

I soon found out, however, that responsibilities came along with having my own place. We were all expected to do chores, and I was *very* unhappy to hear that! I was not used to cleaning anything myself because I never had to lift a finger while I was growing up. My two sisters did all of the cooking and cleaning since my mother worked part-time. And my grandmother always had a cleaning lady so I never had to help out when I visited her either.

Odessa and Rosalie were used to cleaning, so I would try to get them to do my share of the chores. The only thing I didn't mind was grocery shopping. But, there was no way I was about to clean the bathroom or even fold laundry. I do like everything to be nice, and I like to tell people how I want things, but I don't want to do any of it myself. With this attitude of mine, the personal care attendants immediately pegged me as a spoiled prima donna, and said I was "born with a silver spoon in my mouth." I became quite unpopular with the staff.

XII

I was very happy living with Rosalie and Odessa. We had many good times together, and we treated each other like family. I was considerably more content with them than with my real family. Any problems that we did encounter involved our personal care attendants, and they were often quite serious ones.

To say that we were mistreated by some of our attendants would be a gross understatement. At times, their behavior was inhumane, and the fact that it was intentional made it more horrible. The three of us were in a very difficult and vulnerable position. We were dependent on these people for our physical well-being, yet we would suffer immensely if we ever angered them.

I personally had very specific needs, yet one of the attendants did not want me telling her how to take care of me. On one occasion, she decided she wasn't listening to me anymore. Instead of administering my own medication, she gave me some of hers. It put me to sleep for an entire week. When people from United Cerebral Palsy questioned her about my condition, she lied and said that I had the flu.

This mean-spirited woman treated us terribly. However, we knew that if we spoke up and complained to someone at United Cerebral Palsy, we would pay the consequences. We felt trapped, and forced to accept many atrocities because we were afraid of retaliation. If we made her angry enough, she would leave me in bed all day, and then think of ways to aggravate Odessa and Rosalie.

A few times we became so frightened that we called the police. However, we didn't get any results. Since there was only one attendant on duty at a time, there were no witnesses to our mistreatment. Therefore, when confronted, she would deny any wrongdoing. She was a master at covering up her actions, and in the process made it look like we didn't know what we were talking about. She basically portrayed us as idiots who were just imagining things.

For some reason, she immensely enjoyed terrifying Rosalie. On a number of occasions, she would tell us that someone was outside our window. We *would* see a person staring in, but didn't know it was actually her girlfriend. Rosalie would be scared to death, and get herself so upset that she would end up having to go to the hospital. The attendant seemed to find this whole deception extremely amusing. Once again, if one of us called the police, she would convince them that it never happened.

An ongoing situation with this woman eventually became unbearable though. There is a limit to what anyone can endure, and this went far beyond it. Quite often, she had her lesbian girlfriend visit her in our apartment. Unfortunately, watching Odessa, Rosalie, and me get undressed became entertainment for them. We were not only furious, but tremendously disappointed knowing that someone who was supposed to be caring for us could do something so wretched. But, even worse, the degradation and humiliation we experienced was beyond description. Our life was becoming a nightmare.

Finally, one day from hell brought everything to a head. The personal care attendant sat Rosalie in the Hoyer lift, and put her into the shower. She turned the water on and left her there unattended. She refused to get me out of bed. Then she purposely dropped Odessa on the floor, and left her there, too. All of a sudden, the woman became frightened and ran out of the apartment, leaving the three of us in a terrible predicament. Fortunately, I was able to reach a phone. I called United Cerebral Palsy who contacted Kevin Randall, one of the senior counselors there.

Although Kevin was busy at the time caring for three male residents, he immediately dropped everything. He put the men in a van, and came right over to help us. When he arrived, he was appalled by what he saw. After helping each one of us out of our specific dilemma, he called the head supervisor at United Cerebral Palsy. He strongly suggested calling the police in order to keep the two lesbians from coming back into our home. Kevin then stayed with us until other coverage arrived. Meanwhile, the police found our attendant and arrested her. She had been abusing us for five months, and was going to be punished for her actions at last.

If your support staff is hired through an agency, it's very difficult to let them go. Often the attendant's word will be taken over yours. Even if you are believed, you don't always get results. The agency tends to cover up any improprieties in order to protect their reputation. It took another five months and about six separate meetings with United Cerebral Palsy to convince them that we were living in unacceptable conditions, but we persevered – and the offending worker was finally fired.

XIII

Choosing personal care attendants is even more complicated than selecting an apartment. There are numerous variables to consider including – but not limited to – competency, reliability, compassion, honesty, and very importantly, compatibility. In some ways, the relationship between client and caregiver is similar to a marriage. If you can't get along with each other, it's just not going to work.

Start by interviewing as many prospective attendants as possible, and remember that first impressions are not always accurate. Naturally, everyone shows their best face at an interview since they're trying to land a job. In truth, it's extremely difficult to select the perfect caregiver because until you actually live and work with someone, you're not going to know if the two of you are a good match. No matter how well the interview goes, only after you experience that person in your life, can you tell what he or she is really like.

Be prepared with your questions for the interviews. I always like to ask why the person is interested in this type of work. In addition, I want to know what the term "self-direction" means to them, and make sure the answer matches my own personal definition. Ask for a resume and check references. Don't forget, for your own safety, a criminal background check is an absolute must.

During the interview process, you must emphasize your individualized needs. Make it known that first and foremost, those needs must be met. This is the time to make all expectations as clear as possible. If hired, the attendant cannot decide what she *thinks* you need. Those decisions are completely up to you and you alone. It's all about what you're comfortable with whether she agrees or not. These are not her choices to make. She must not only provide for the necessities of your life but also your personal preferences. Be specific! If you like to go for long walks or want to go shopping at the mall, or if you like to have makeup applied every day, she must be willing to accommodate your wishes.

While you are interviewing, you will find that everyone is not willing to perform each and every duty. Most likely, you will need to hire a few people in order to cover a variety of jobs. The attendant who takes care of your personal hygiene might not be a good cook – and the cook may not be capable of helping you with your banking needs. You may even have to hire other staff specifically to do the cleaning. If so, make it clear that you expect them to treat your house like they do their own. If they don't leave dirty dishes and unmade beds at their place, then they should understand that it won't be acceptable at yours.

In my experience, I have found that some caregivers look down on you. They don't give you the respect you deserve, and do not consider you their equal. Be firm! Remember, you are the boss and they are working for you.

It is imperative that you hire people who look at you and see a man or a woman, not just a challenging physical condition. They must be willing to give you the tools that you need to lead your best life possible. Although they must be aware of the specific assistance that you need, they must also take into consideration that you are an adult, and want to be treated like one. Personally, although I like to be pampered a bit, I abhor being overly protected and smothered. I don't like people to go to extremes with me. Give me what I need, but realize that I am a grown woman. I don't want to be told what to do. My body may not be flawless, but my brain is just fine. I'm the one – and the only one – who knows *best* what's best for me!

Although attendants spend many hours with you and take physical care of you, they don't know what it's like living your life. Sometimes a caregiver may make a suggestion "in your best interest," and you might disagree with it. If that happens, say "no" to the suggestion and stand your ground. If you have compassionate attendants, they will defer to your wishes. I must tell you, however, that if you are unfortunate enough to have an intolerant one, he or she might make you pay for your assertiveness. This has happened to me. I have personally found that the word "no" coming from a client is often the worst word for some attendants to accept. Depending on the individual involved and the circumstances, I have, at times, had to put up with some pretty unpleasant conditions until it was possible to make a staff change.

If you do have an unsatisfactory situation with an attendant, you must speak up and tell someone. If it is a serious problem such as some type of abuse or impropriety, or neglect, contact Adult Protective Services or the police. My strong suggestion is to go somewhere safe to make the phone call, so that you can report your complaints privately. You don't want the offender to overhear your conversation. Hopefully, the police will believe you. Then they can remove the attendant from your home and protect you from danger.

It really doesn't matter if you hire a personal care attendant through an agency or on your own. Either way, there is no guarantee that you will find suitable help. Life is life, and people are people. There are good and bad people everywhere and hiring through an agency does not necessarily assure you a positive experience. No matter how many times you have to hire and fire, keep searching until you find someone you feel is right for you.

Even if you do find an appropriate attendant, the turnover rate is relatively high in this particular field of work. I have had more caregivers than I care to count, with the shortest stay only six months and the longest three years. The monetary compensation is poor and the benefits are substandard. It is a time-consuming position, and can be physically demanding, as well. Combine all of those factors, and it's understandable why some employees may burn out after a short time on the job.

For a number of possible reasons, you may find out later that the attendant you hired was not the best choice, after all. It could be that you get along wonderfully together, but actually have become too close. That can interfere with the employee/employer relationship. Too much familiarity can cause you to lose your perspective. If problems do develop, you may be uncomfortable addressing them because you feel more like a friend than a supervisor. But you have to hold your ground. If the caregiver is unwilling to do what you request, you must find someone who will. And, of course, if you feel like you are not receiving proper care, or if you are left alone and unattended, terminate the worker immediately.

XIV

Despite my family's doubts about my moving out, my mother and Earl visited me often in that first apartment of mine. As the years passed however, their visits became less frequent. They were bothered by the fact that I preferred living with my roommates instead of them. They didn't understand why I would choose a life with virtual strangers over my own family.

On the other hand, my real father and his wife Irene continued to visit me and have me to their house throughout the years. I looked forward to seeing my dad as much as I did when I was a little girl.

Over time, I also came to realize that my closeness to people of other races disturbed my mother, stepfather, and siblings. They are all racists. I have very strong beliefs about accepting people regardless of their color or race, and they disagree vehemently with my views. They are extremely prejudiced, and have made it abundantly clear that they do not like many of my friends. My siblings have gone so far as to accuse me of loving my "nigger friends" more than I love them. They should know that my love is not dependent on the color of a person's skin. It has to do solely with respect and caring, and nobody can change my feelings about that. If someone cares for me and shows me respect, I will care for them and respect them in return. It's that simple. Can't my family see that I have friends who have cared for me and respected me more than they ever did?

Sadly, a person's family can sometimes prove to be her own worst enemy. Quite often, my family has chosen to make themselves unavailable to me when I really needed them. So, when they weren't there for me, out of sheer necessity, I turned to others for help. And frankly, it never mattered to me if the people who helped me were black, white, purple, or blue.

XV

Something else that really threw my family for a loop was when I decided to get married. I met Neil Kevin Jerome Speciner at a United Cerebral Palsy day program called The Place when I was 20 years old. He was also one of their clients and had many physical challenges of his own. We had been dating for five years, so it should not have been a surprise to anyone that we had long-term plans. When we announced that we were getting married, however, we were bombarded with objections from everybody! They all weighed in with an opinion, and not one of them was encouraging. For various reasons, everyone tried to convince us to reconsider our decision.

Neil's mother was a strict Catholic, so she was distressed to learn that I was a Methodist. She questioned him repeatedly about whether he was certain that he wanted to marry me. Even on our wedding day, she pulled Neil aside to ask him one more time if he was sure! My own mother couldn't quite imagine what I was thinking, and didn't understand my desire to experience married life. I was in love with Neil but since she did not view us in the same way she viewed other men and women, this was beyond her comprehension.

I mistakenly assumed that my mother would prefer that I marry Neil rather than just live with him. Years earlier, my sister ran away and moved in with her boyfriend before they were married. This unfortunate incident caused a terrible rift, and much grief, in our family. My mother refused to speak to her for years. In addition to marrying Neil because I loved him, I also wanted to keep peace in our family and not upset my mother again. Although getting married would be a financial hardship and would require changing residential agencies, I believed it was the respectable thing to do for my mother. I had learned from my sister's experience, and didn't want to repeat her mistake. It wasn't until years later, that my mother admitted to me that it wouldn't have mattered to her, at all, if we had lived together. Once again she made it clear that, in her eyes, nothing about me or my life was the same as my sister's.

The financial ramifications of getting married, though severe, would not sway us from our decision either. My father had to remove me from life and health insurance policies because Neil would now be considered the head of our household. My father even argued that I had a disability, but his reasoning fell on deaf ears. The insurance company would not budge on its decision. Also, the amount of money I was receiving from SSI would be split in half between Neil and me once we were married. In addition, the Social Security Disability Income that Neil had been collecting since his father's death would also be withdrawn after our marriage. Representatives from Social Security actually told us that we would be better off financially if we just lived together. That way, we wouldn't lose so much money. It seemed as though we were being penalized for doing the appropriate thing.

During our courtship, both Neil and I lived in homes managed by United Cerebral Palsy. This would prove to be yet another stumbling block in our desire to marry. United Cerebral Palsy informed us that we could no longer remain residential clients of theirs after our marriage. We would be allowed to stay in their day program, but if we insisted on getting married, we would have to make other living arrangements.

The head of United Cerebral Palsy didn't think marriage was a good idea "for our kind of people," and tried to talk us out of our decision. According to him, we didn't have the same feelings or needs as other people, and we certainly shouldn't have a desire for a sexual relationship. He did his best to change our minds, but he failed.

In the midst of all this turmoil, I needed hip and back surgery. It was during my stay at Montebello Hospital that we actually came upon a solution. Through a kind social worker there, we discovered an agency called Making Choices for

Independent Living. If Neil and I became clients of MCIL, we could get married and live together in housing provided by them. Our transfer from United Cerebral Palsy to Making Choices for Independent Living took about one year, but Neil and I could finally move ahead with our wedding plans.

XVI

Like most brides-to-be, my matron of honor and I handled the majority of the details and preparations for the big day. However, Neil was adamant about personally securing the marriage license. It was something he really wanted to do on his own, so I agreed to let him take care of it. As all brides know, anything you can delegate to someone else is a tremendous help. I was more than happy to relinquish that small but important detail to Neil.

And so, while I was busy inviting our 200 guests, making arrangements for the reception, and gown shopping for my bridesmaids and me, I never gave the marriage license another thought. I asked my two sisters Janice and Jodel to be my bridesmaids, and my girlfriend Joanne to be my matron of honor. Neil's best man was William, a school friend, and his ushers were my sisters' husbands. The ceremony was to be held at a Methodist church on Harford Road, and the Holiday Inn in Towson was booked for the reception. Our wedding date was set for October 30, 1983. Everything was falling into place – or so I thought.

On the evening before the wedding, I was elated as I arrived at the church for the rehearsal. I felt confident that all details had been attended to, and now it was time to relax and enjoy the wondrous day that we had planned. Neil was feeling good, too, and very proud of himself for getting our marriage license. It was not an easy task for him due to his physical challenges. So, he felt a great sense of accomplishment knowing he had succeeded.

As the minister skimmed over our license, a glaring mistake caught his eye. He privately informed us that the license was valid only in Baltimore City, and the church where we were getting married was in Baltimore County. We were stunned! The license was useless! As we began to realize the enormity of our situation, a nightmare seemed to be unfolding. We had 200 guests coming to a wedding the next day that couldn't take place. Neil was terribly disappointed in himself and embarrassed, but I was beginning to feel angry with him. He had one responsibility – just one – and he blew it! All the planning, all the hours, the money – was all of it completely for nothing?

Fortunately, while we were escalating into a panic, the minister was devising a plan to salvage our wedding. Neil and I listened carefully as he explained what we needed to do the next day. Only the three of us would know about this unfortunate snag and its solution.

October 30, 1983 had arrived at last! I felt glorious in my wedding gown, and I remember thinking how strikingly handsome Neil looked in his tuxedo with the gray cummerbund. I was happy, and crying, and nervous all at the same time. This was our special day. A day when our identity would be outside the box of Jacquie and Neil with physical challenges in wheelchairs. On this spectacular day, we would simply be Jacquie and Neil, bride and groom – soon to become husband and wife!

We had arranged for a van from Making Choices for Independent Living to pick us up and transport us to the church. It arrived late that morning, but we didn't let it diminish our excitement. We knew everyone would wait for us!

When we finally arrived at the church, another handsome gentleman greeted me! My biological father was ready to walk me down the aisle. I couldn't have been happier! The man I had loved dearly since birth was escorting me directly to the man I fell in love with and was ready to marry. After my father formally presented me to Neil, the kind-hearted minister began our wedding ceremony.

It was a lovely service, with all of the traditional music, readings, and "repeat after me's" like most other weddings. We just never said those well-known words – "I do!" After we rolled back up the aisle, and greeted everyone in the receiving line, we directed them on to the Holiday Inn.

As soon as the last of the guests departed from the church, Neil and I got back into the van, and the minister started his car. His plan was in motion! Our driver took us over the county line into the city, and pulled into a gas station. When the minister arrived, he climbed into our van, and had us repeat our vows. This time we got to say, "I do." There, in the MCIL van, in the parking lot of a gas station, he pronounced us man and wife. We were now legally married!

No one else knew about our marriage license problem, so when we finally arrived at the reception, everyone wanted to know what took us so long. People were quite astonished when we told them where we had been! Word about our detour was spreading quickly through the crowd as Neil and I were being introduced for the first time in public as Mr. and Mrs. Speciner!

We had a wonderful time at the reception with so many of our friends and family members! I love crowds, and I love being the center of attention, so every minute was exhilarating for me. I felt more special than I ever had before.

When the reception ended, I went up to the room we had reserved at the Holiday Inn to get ready for my new husband. Neil decided to give me a little privacy first, so he said he would hang out in the hotel bar for about an hour and a half. His roommate and two attendants went with him. After a couple of hours, I became upset and impatient for Neil to return – and finally fell asleep. Obviously, Neil was enjoying himself, and was not watching the clock. While the hours were slipping away, he was not only oblivious to the time, but also his bar bill. He managed to go over our set budget, which my father had to address with him the next morning! He was not off to a good start – with me or my Dad!

Neil finally came up to our room at 2:00 a.m. I was angry, and let him know it, but he did apologize and convinced me that his actions were not intentional. He won me over, and I am happy to say that we eventually had the wedding night I had always hoped for.

XVII

I adore being in the spotlight, so I was thrilled when United Cerebral Palsy wanted to air the videotape of our wedding during their national telethon. Since they would not allow Neil and me to remain in their residential program after we were married, it seemed rather hypocritical that they wanted to showcase our special event – but we said we'd allow it. Naturally, it was contrived to make their agency look highly progressive and appealing to the public. They even requested that Neil and I appear live on the telethon. The idea was to portray United Cerebral Palsy in a positive light, boost donations to the agency, and enhance its reputation. I love the media, and although I was upset by their attitude toward our marriage, Neil and I agreed to make an appearance on the show. It was a marvelous experience, and we felt like pampered celebrities.

XVIII

Neil and I started our married life in an apartment with just the two of us and our attendants. Michael, a counselor with MCIL, helped us immensely during those early days. He located apartments for us, and then helped us secure funding so we could afford them. Michael came through for us time and time again. He even counseled us during our first two years of marriage. The work that he did for us was much more than a job to Michael. He visited Neil and me many times, often bringing along his wife and children. His wife helped us, too, and even learned how to take me to the bathroom. We loved those visits, and looked forward to the time we spent with this unique man and his wonderful family.

When Neil and I were in the process of hiring personal care attendants, Michael would make sure he was available to be present at the interviews. I didn't require quite the amount of physical care as Neil did. So sometimes we shared an attendant, and other times we each had our own – a male for Neil and a female for me.

One exceptional attendant who cared for both Neil and me was Janet. She came from Jamaica, leaving her family behind. She worked with us for two years. Her seven year old son would visit her here for two weeks in the summertime. We looked forward to having him around, too. Janet was a marvelous cook, and I thought her Jamaican food was absolutely delicious. She took excellent care of both of us, and I truly loved her.

Although she had occasional breaks, she basically had a 24 hour a day position. However, her salary was just $50 a day, and she only received one paycheck per month. Half of her pay came from Neil's Medical Assistance, and the other half from mine. To make matters worse, Medical Assistance stopped every six months for review and to be verified. Eventually, Janet's salary was cut in half. Twenty-five dollars a day to take complete, physical care of two people is preposterous. She had been sending money to Jamaica for her son's care, and trying to live off what was left of that measly salary. Eventually, it became financially impossible, and to our dismay and hers, she had to leave us. Neil and I completely understood, but were sad and disappointed to see her go.

Our next attendant was also hired with our Medical Assistance funds. We experienced many problems with this woman. She was from Africa, and knew nothing about refrigeration. When I saw meat setting on the kitchen counter, I told her to throw it away, and explained to her that meat must be kept in the refrigerator. She argued with me about it assuming that since I had cerebral palsy, I didn't know what I was saying. Neil and I both became violently ill with diarrhea from eating contaminated food, and she would leave us dirty because her husband said that would teach us a lesson. I finally called my mother and told her we had been sick for days. She came over with a fresh supply of food, and threw out what we had. A whole month's worth of groceries was wasted. My mother was livid, and gave that attendant two things – a piece of her mind and no mercy!

When someone from United Cerebral Palsy came to check on us, she found our clothes soiled with waste and hidden in the closet. These also had to be disposed of. In addition, we found out that the woman lied about not having another job. According to the Medical Assistance agreement, an attendant receives free room, board, and utilities, and in exchange agrees not to work anywhere else. She had broken that agreement. Thankfully, the attendant was fired, and we were relieved to see the last of her.

On a more positive note, one of our attendants was so dedicated that, despite her degenerative eye disease, she took a bus from Washington, DC to our place in Baltimore every weekend. It was not easy for Sharon to make that trip but Neil and I were very grateful that she did. She was conscientious about her work and she made sure everything was always clean. She never once complained about the physical care she had to give us either.

Sharon often completed the unfinished work of our other attendants, but she didn't like when that took time away from her own duties.

What we enjoyed most about Sharon though was that she was a tremendous amount of fun. Neil and I always looked forward to her arrival because when she came for the weekend, we knew we'd be doing something special. When Sharon was with us, we were constantly on the go, and rarely at home. Sometimes, she would bring her children and we'd all spend the day at the Baltimore Harborplace. Or, Sharon got on the mobility van with us to attend live performances at Merriwether Post Pavilion in Columbia, Maryland. We loved that she was willing to travel around town with us and go on so many outings.

Occasionally, Sharon would be late, but she possessed so many positive qualities that I was willing to overlook that single flaw once in awhile. Because of her macular degeneration, it was not easy for her to get to us, and I took that into consideration. But, not my husband… Neil was not so forgiving and made a major issue out of it. He began yelling at Sharon whenever she wasn't on time. She resented being reprimanded, and eventually quit because of Neil's complaining.

I was so angry with him for spoiling the wonderful relationship we had with Sharon. She was kind-hearted and good to us, and I really loved her. I couldn't believe Neil had driven her away.

My husband did get along well with Patty however. She was initially Neil's attendant when he was a resident at Rosewood. After we were married and had transferred to MCIL, Patty worked with both of us. She was able to do something for me that no other attendant could. Because of her past history with Neil, she could entertain me with hilarious stories about him during their time together at Rosewood. Patty could really keep me laughing with her humorous anecdotes – all at Neil's expense.

I suppose if I did an actual head count, I've most likely had more challenging experiences with personal care attendants than positive ones. But I have had the good fortune to know some very unique people through the years – people who have touched my life and my heart.

Brian is one of those exceptional individuals. He worked with Neil and me through United Cerebral Palsy. He was amazing! Whatever needed to be done, he did it willingly with no complaints. He cleaned; he cooked; and he kept both our place and us spotless. Brian and Neil hung out and watched wrestling matches together. They thoroughly enjoyed each other's company – but then United Cerebral Palsy had to interfere. The agency doesn't like to see attendants and clients become too friendly because they think it will spoil the clients. So, after an exemplary nine year work record, United Cerebral Palsy decided to make things difficult for Brian. Suddenly, he was required to take a test on medications – a test that was not mandatory before. Now, all of a sudden, it became a priority.

In addition to this obstacle, other staff members began to tell lies about Brian, and United Cerebral Palsy believed them. Brian felt betrayed. He really thought that after nine years, the agency should have trusted him. Neil and I could always count on Brian, and we desperately wanted him to stay. But the lack of respect United Cerebral Palsy showed to him caused him to resign. It was a sorry day when Brian left us.

XIX

When both a husband and a wife have physical challenges, there are countless details to be handled on a daily basis. Sometimes, it is scheduling appointments with doctors or making sure prescriptions are filled. Other days, it may be arranging transportation or planning menus. And quite often, dealing with staff issues that come up takes a tremendous amount of time. Initially, I wanted to take care of all these things myself.

I realize now that I made a mistake by assuming responsibility for every aspect of our daily lives. It was my decision, and Neil readily agreed to it, but I would never put myself in that position again. I handled just about everything for both of us, and made sure that Neil had whatever he needed. It seemed like a good idea at first, but it would have been much better for our relationship if we had shared all the responsibilities. The way I had taken over, did not foster an equal partnership in our marriage. Neil would have benefited from a more important role in our life together. It would have been better for both of us.

I know this because Neil was most proud of himself when he held a job through supported employment with United Cerebral Palsy. His salary may have been small but his sense of accomplishment was huge. It meant a lot to Neil and really improved his self-image to know he was providing for me. It also gave him a good reason to get up in the morning and put on nice clothes. Our relationship was strongest and we were both happier when he was working. When he lost that job, through no fault of his own, our marriage began to suffer.

Neil had what I like to call "memory select syndrome." He would often pick and choose what to remember whenever it suited him. He liked to remember pleasant things – for instance, something special that made me happy. That was all well and good, but it's what he chose to forget that caused trouble. Our worst arguments involved this particular syndrome of his.

If Neil and I had a problem with an attendant, we would discuss it, but then *I* would have to confront the person. This was because all of a sudden, Neil "wouldn't remember" what the problem was and would act like nothing was wrong. He would sometimes go so far as to contradict me in front of the attendant, and say that there wasn't a problem at all. Even if someone hurt one of us, and I reported it, sometimes Neil would lie and deny that it happened. Ultimately, this made *me* look like the liar and seem like a nasty woman. Although I was speaking for both of us, Neil came out looking like the perfect gentleman. He always wanted everyone to like him, and didn't mind at all that I looked stupid and became the heavy. It was something that we argued about frequently.

Neil was perfectly content letting me control our affairs, unless something went wrong. If he didn't like the way I handled a situation, he would have no problem making me feel inadequate and look like a fool. It didn't occur to him to spare my feelings, or take into consideration that I was carrying a heavy load for the two of us.

To Neil's credit however, he would do the best he could to be supportive if he knew someone was mistreating me. Unfortunately, he didn't always know. There were times when I chose not to share that kind of information with him.

One of his attendants named Rob used me as his play toy for about a year and a half. He was utterly disgusting and always had a horrendous case of body odor. He knew I despised him, yet took advantage of every available opportunity to rape me. He literally made me nauseous, and I vomited every time he finished with me. Although this happened over and over again, I was afraid to tell anyone including Neil. I didn't think people would believe me. As I have said, often an attendant's word would be taken over a client's. I also liked the other attendants we had at the time, and it was possible that if they knew the truth, they might have attacked

Rob and been arrested themselves. I didn't want to cause trouble for them either, so consequently, I kept quiet.

Fortunately, there are the personal care attendants who go above and beyond their job descriptions and required responsibilities. Amelia was one of those rare individuals. Taking care of Neil and me was not just a job to her. Amelia truly cared about us, and it showed in her actions. She let me cook with her which took a great deal of patience on her part. And if the van didn't come for me, she still managed to get me where I needed to go. Even Amelia's boyfriend Shakey helped us out. He would lift me into his car, and take me to the grocery store. Amelia often included Neil and me in her own family's special events. For a year and a half, she was a very positive influence in our lives.

Sadly, I have since learned that Amelia suffered from stomach cancer, and had been on medical leave for three or four years. I received word that she passed away early in February 2006. As a personal care attendant, she was one of the best. As a friend, she was a wonderful treasure.

Another of our personal care attendants who is still very special to me is Sary. Neil and I met her through our next door neighbor Tony. Sary was actually Tony's attendant but eventually, with the help of her girlfriend Dee, took care of all three of us. Neil and I were a handful considering our physical challenges, plus Tony was paralyzed from an automobile accident. Together we were a tremendous responsibility. After his accident, Tony's wife couldn't cope with his condition and left him. At that time, he became a client of MCIL and Sary was hired to work for him.

Despite the unfortunate turn of events in his life, Tony never lost his positive attitude. He continued to live life to the fullest. He never let his paralysis discourage him. He was an accomplished artist, and was successful in selling his paintings. Tony was a true inspiration to many people, and a marvelous role model for Neil and me.

It was our good fortune that Tony agreed to share Sary with us. She was a gem, and she cared for us like we were her own family. Sary did some remarkable things for us that no other attendant had done – things she was not obligated to do. She was hired only to clean us and the house, cook, and get us up in the morning. However, she saw to it that we enjoyed life, too, and made sure we did a lot of socializing. Although she didn't get paid for it, she would take us to bull roasts and to the movies. If the mobility van didn't show up, even though Neil was 300 pounds, she would lift us into a cab to get us wherever we wanted to go.

Neil and I were so content and happy for the year and a half that Sary was with us. But, once again, the paychecks from Medical Assistance caused trouble for us. Although Sary should have been paid once a month, the checks were often two or three months late. That was totally unacceptable. She could not make ends meet. She couldn't pay her bills, or tend to her own personal needs. Sometimes, she couldn't even buy herself essentials, like soap. When her situation got really bad, Neil and I bought her food, and gave her extra money at the beginning of the month.

Sary's pay was only $50 a day to care for both of us, but since she wasn't even receiving that, she gradually began doing less and less for us. Although we were like family to her, Sary stopped cleaning us. We certainly couldn't blame her for getting tired of working and not being compensated. Unfortunately, our personal care continued to decline.

Despite the fact that Neil and I hired Sary, United Cerebral Palsy stepped in at this point and fired her. They didn't realize she wasn't getting paid, and they accused her of abuse because we were dirty. I couldn't believe it! United Cerebral Palsy rarely helped when we needed them, yet took control away from us when we didn't want them to. Abuse? Compared to what I had endured many times in the past, I certainly didn't consider being dirty abuse. I had survived so much worse.

Although Sary was forced to leave, we parted ways on amicable terms. After she was gone, we knew if we needed her, we could still call on her to help us out occasionally. I wish I could see Sary again someday, and I will always love her. She had a difficult life herself, but she did everything she could to make ours pleasant.

An incident that had a lasting impact on Neil and me involved another male caregiver. This man often drank alcohol and had sexual relations with my female attendant right in our own home. Sadly, he switched his attention from her to me one day. It didn't matter to him that I was on the bedpan, and also on the telephone with my grandmother at the time. He took advantage of my complete helplessness and raped me. Neil was in the living room when the man came out of my bedroom with his pants still open. When Neil questioned him, he gave the excuse that he forgot to zip up after using the bathroom.

A few minutes later, one of our bus drivers came to the door with some Christmas presents for us. She came into my bedroom to visit me, and could sense that I was upset. When she asked me though, I couldn't tell her because the man was still in the apartment. She left without knowing what was wrong. When my attacker finally went home, he left a stove burner lit underneath of a pot. Although this could have been disastrous, it actually turned out to be fortunate for me. Later, a neighbor saw smoke through our window and called 911. When the police arrived, I told them about the rape. When Neil heard my story, he was outraged, but comforted me as best he could.

In typical fashion, the accused offender tried to defend himself by saying that I was out of my mind, and didn't know what I was talking about. However, Neil had gone with me to the hospital where evidence was collected and the rape was confirmed. The man was arrested and sent to jail for three years.

Although Neil knew in his heart that the rape was not my fault, he simply could not cope with what had happened to me. He greatly resented what the man had done, and couldn't seem to move beyond it. He even became fixated on the fact that I could not have children – something that he had accepted years before. Unfortunately, our marriage and relationship started a downward spiral after that.

At first we didn't get along very well with our personal care attendant Jeremy, but eventually he became like family to us. He was a lot closer to Neil but he often cared for both of us. In fact, if my female attendant was off, Jeremy was capable of dressing me and taking me to the bathroom. He came to us from Temporary Healthcare, and was really fun to have around. He was a great kidder - always making us laugh.

Our only problem with Jeremy was when he became romantically involved with my caregiver. First of all, Neil and I didn't think it was appropriate for them to carry on their love affair right in our apartment. But I later realized that I was actually jealous of their relationship. At this point, Neil and I were having marital problems. Our own relationship wasn't going well, and to put it delicately, my physical needs were not being met. To see our attendants enjoying themselves so much, simply underscored what I didn't have.

Eventually however, they began having disagreements with each other, and would put me in the middle. They'd want me to relay their messages to each other – tell her this, and tell him that. It caused a lot of tension for all of us. In order to avoid such problems, it's better to have only one attendant on duty at a time. We learned that lesson the hard way.

XX

Neil had always been somewhat flirtatious with the ladies, but I was able to put up with his behavior as long as it remained innocent. However, after the rape, in addition to experiencing drastic mood swings, he was starting to pay too much attention to one of my female attendants. He began giving her money causing some of my checks to bounce. Things between them progressed to the point where I realized that Neil was cheating on me with my own caregiver. Of course, he refused to admit the truth. However, he didn't have to, after I witnessed it firsthand for myself. Neil had sex with this woman while I was in the room with them. Unbelievably, he continued to lie and denied that it happened until I told him that I had actually seen the two of them together. It was the last straw, and I informed him that he had to get out and find another place to live. After twelve years of marriage, I wanted a divorce.

Many people were surprised by our separation. They couldn't believe it. What they saw was Neil's intelligence, and how well he treated me on special occasions. And they knew that I was very protective of him. Everything looked fine on the surface, but underneath, our problems were more serious than anyone would have guessed. I still loved Neil, and even after he moved out, I was concerned for his well-being. I checked to make sure he ate well, and I let his weekend attendant do Neil's laundry at my place. I allowed Neil to come over, too, but there was no way he was going to live with me anymore.

Our relationship continued in this vein for about a year. We were always in touch and saw each other frequently. We had our disagreements but we remained close friends throughout our separation.

XXI

If Neil was one thing, he was hard-headed. When he made up his mind about something, that was it. No reconsidering his decision. No turning back. I personally attribute that to the fact that he was born on July 16th under the sign of the Cancer. He also had trouble choosing a common sense approach over an approach that would attain him instant gratification. Unfortunately, these characteristics of his would indirectly play a role in his demise.

Neil and I each had a device called a Hoyer lift. The lift is a bulky machine that consists of a metal frame and chains connected to a sling which is under the user. It transferred us from one place to another. For example, it would lift us from our wheelchairs and lower us into bed or the bathtub. Neil was a big man – not tall – but approximately 300 pounds. I told Neil that considering his size, he needed a heavyweight Hoyer, but of course he knew better and ordered a lightweight model. This was an unwise decision on his part.

One evening, Neil was invited to a party in the apartment upstairs from him. He knew it was always a good idea to go to the bathroom before leaving home. He should have used the urinal that night before he left for the party, but he was so anxious to get going, that he decided not to take the time. His attendant even suggested it, but Neil refused. The choice he made that night proved to be a bigger mistake than anyone could have ever predicted.

While Neil was at the party, he urinated in the Hoyer. By the time he got back down to his own apartment, the Hoyer sling was sliding down out of its proper position. The combination of Neil's weight and the slippery sling caused the lift to tip over onto its side. Neil ended up with a broken femur, and was taken to the hospital emergency room.

XXII

What took place after that will remain a mystery to me forever. Neil was not unconscious. He only had a broken leg, so I know he would have told the ambulance attendant and someone at the hospital that he was allergic to morphine. Ordinarily, when a person goes to the hospital, one question is repeated over and over again: Are you allergic to any medications? Neil was perfectly aware of his medical history. Over the two day period that he was in the hospital, I know he would have told a number of people about his allergy. So, I will never understand why they gave him morphine. I often wonder if no one believed him. Was it another case of someone thinking that because Neil was in a wheelchair, he didn't know what he was talking about? Sadly, an overdose of morphine left Neil brain dead.

At the time of Neil's accident, he was angry with me. Therefore, when he was admitted to the hospital, he listed my sister Janice as a contact. So, she was the one who was informed about the hospital's dreadful error – instead of me.

Shortly before that, I had had an accident of my own. As I was being taken off the bedpan in my wheelchair, I heard a loud crack. I wound up in the emergency room with a broken femur, too. Therefore, when I finally found out about Neil's condition, we both had broken bones.

I was living with a woman named Mrs. Gibson at this time, and she called the hospital to check on Neil's condition for me. She had the misfortune of speaking with an extremely rude nurse. Mrs. Gibson began crying while she was on the phone, and I wanted to know what was happening. She put the phone on speaker mode, and I could not believe what I was hearing. The nurse began making awful comments about Neil not being a worthwhile person. She couldn't have been more wrong though. He *did* contribute to society by working in supported employment.

She even insinuated that it was really no big deal that Neil was brain dead. It was excruciatingly painful for me to hear such scathing remarks about him. She didn't know anything about him, yet she made a rash judgment based solely on his appearance. As long as I live, I will never forget that very emotional phone call and the insensitivity of the nurse as she delivered such devastating news to us. But I knew then that it was time for me to go say goodbye to Neil.

Mrs. Gibson and I went to the hospital as soon as we could. When we got off the elevator, we encountered another ill-tempered nurse. I suppose since my femur was broken and I was on a stretcher, it was understandable that she thought I was a patient. But regardless, her nasty tone when she barked, "Where does she belong?" was completely uncalled for and inappropriate. In no uncertain terms, I angrily informed her that I was not a patient, that I was Neil Speciner's wife, and that I was there to see my husband one last time. I made it distinctly clear that she had better not mess with me. I was already furious enough by the medical mistreatment Neil had received and the revolting phone conversation I had earlier. I was in no mood for anymore aggravation. Neil and I both deserved to be treated with the respect and dignity that this unfortunate situation called for.

As I entered Neil's room, I was aware of what I was going to have to do. He had a living will, and I knew precisely what it said. As difficult and heartbreaking as it would be, I knew deep inside I had to abide by his wishes. And so, after spending some last private moments with my husband, I did the hardest thing there is to do in this life. With a heavy heart, I turned off the machine that was keeping him alive. Neil died two days later on August 2nd at the age of 47.

We didn't have the best marriage, but I loved Neil and mourned his passing. It has been over ten years now, and although most days I am fine, holidays are still extremely hard for me. Neil loved all holidays, but particularly Christmas. He had happy childhood memories of Christmases with his family. It was his absolute favorite time of the year. I get extremely depressed each Christmas, thinking about Neil and how unnecessary his death was. He only had a broken leg. He should not have died.

XXIII

At the time of Neil's death, I was still legally his wife. Our divorce had not been finalized yet. So, this made it possible for me to file a lawsuit against the hospital.

The hospital did, in fact, admit wrongdoing. They acknowledged that an overdose of morphine was indeed the cause of Neil's death. Not only did someone administer morphine to him despite his allergy, just one dose was written on his medical chart. The fact is that he received a total of three doses, but the other two were never recorded. Three doses of morphine are more than any adult – with or without cerebral palsy, allergic to the drug or not – could tolerate. The amount of morphine given to Neil would have killed anyone.

I won a wrongful death suit against the hospital, and the settlement I received would provide for my long-term care. As Neil's legal widow, I had a right to the money. Nevertheless, this caused enormous turmoil in Neil's family. His three sisters – Barbara, Sue, and Kathy – took me to court in an effort to discredit me and prove that I was incapable of handling the money. Barbara went so far as to lie in court, saying that I had Muscular Dystrophy. To an able-bodied person, this may seem like a minor detail. However, to a person with a specific physical challenge, it is actually insulting to have another challenge put on them that they do not have.

Barbara really had no business getting involved in this situation. She did nothing for her brother when he was alive. It was obvious she was just angry with me and wanted control of Neil's money. His sisters had even taken everything from his apartment. It was becoming a very ugly matter.

In the end, an unlikely ally came to my defense. I will never forget how my mother stood up for me in court. She testified that although she did not agree with all of my decisions or choices in life, she could honestly vouch for the fact that I did my very best for Neil. She knew without a doubt that I did everything I possibly could to make sure Neil had whatever he needed. I have never been more proud of her.

Thankfully, the court ruled in my favor, and so, even though Neil is gone, he is still providing for much of my care. And despite his sisters' accusations that I was unable to handle his money, I am doing just fine. I also know that this is how Neil would have wanted it.

XXIV

I saw a good deal of my biological father until he became sick with colon cancer. All good fathers want to protect their children from unpleasant things. Mine couldn't bear the thought that I would see him suffer and deteriorate during his illness. He wanted to spare me that agony so, to my dismay, I never saw him during the last seven years of his life. When I did finally see him, he was lying in his casket, and he didn't look anything like the man I knew. My father thought in his heart that he was doing the best thing for me, but I would have preferred to see him even though he was sick. At least it would have been an opportunity to spend more time with him. He died in 2000, and to this day, I feel cheated out of those seven years.

Even in death, the two most important men in my life demonstrated their love for me. My father set up a trust that would be sufficient to take care of most of my outside needs. His will stipulates specific things the money can and cannot be used for, but there is plenty set aside for me to live comfortably. The money is not intended to be spent on household items or ordinary, everyday expenses. My SSI pays for those things, including rent and groceries, and my DDA funds pay my attendants' salaries. If I need additional support to help me while I am employed, I may use my trust money. However, those extra support personnel may not be the same people who take care of me at home. I must hire someone entirely new to help me outside my house. I can spend the money that my father left me on any medical bills which are not covered by my insurance. This can include medication, hospital, and ambulance bills. I can also use it for business trips, or to pay a transcriber if I need one to assist me while I take college courses.

It sounds ideal, but there's one enormous problem that really complicates matters for me. I don't have ready access to my own money. My stepbrother Michael, along with my sister Janice, controls every penny that my father left me. To make matters worse, they are most definitely not a "hands on" family. I haven't seen, or even talked to, Michael since my father died in 2000, and he doesn't bother to check with me to see if I need anything either. In fact, he has no communication with me at all, so I really can't depend on him.

Michael is also inconsistent about paying my bills. I had an outstanding charge for an ambulance transport that he kept ignoring. It has taken him as long as four months to pay some of my bills. This is a tremendous worry for me because if I end up with bad credit, I am liable to lose my apartment. Michael is not looking out for my best interests, and if my father knew what was going on, he would be furious. He would be appalled to know that my brother never even acknowledged 10 or 15 phone calls from me requesting a bed! A bed is not a luxury, it is a basic necessity. The trust was set up to make it easy for me to take care of myself – and it's been anything but easy.

It should not be such a hassle for me to get my hands on *my* money. So, I am going to do what I can to rectify this situation as soon as possible. I am planning to have a lawyer change the provisions of my father's will, and take control of my trust away from my siblings. Without a doubt, I expect Michael and Janice to fight me on this. They will say my father set it up this way, and that's how it should stay. But, they are overstepping the boundaries my father would have drawn. They'll also try to say I am not competent to handle my own funds because I used to give money to my attendants if they needed it. However, I will argue that point with them. I realize it was an improper way to use my money, and I've stopped doing that. I am capable of handling my own trust fund, and it is time for them to relinquish the responsibility to me.

When I pass away, the remaining money will pay off any outstanding bills, and the rest will go to my family. I am not particularly anxious to leave them a bundle of money. I'd much rather use it all than leave it to people who have shown so little interest in me. I want to really live this life I have, and utilize the funds available to me while I'm here.

On the other hand, the money I received from Neil's wrongful death suit is much easier for me to access. MCIL has the power of attorney, but they are responsive to my needs and requests. That money is also available for outside use only, but it is attainable within a reasonable amount of time. For example, if I want to go out to dinner, that can be approved with four days notice. Again, medicine not covered by insurance may be paid for with these funds. I can also use this money to take a vacation, and for a clothes shopping trip once a year.

Naturally, I would much rather have Neil and my father still here with me. But, it's comforting to know that even in their absence, they continue to look out for me, and make sure I have what I need to lead my best life possible.

And they will be the *only* men taking care of me financially for the rest of my life. I mean that literally. There will never be anyone else. If I remarried, I would lose every cent of my father's trust and Neil's settlement. My new husband would be considered the head of our household, and my funds would be completely eliminated. I am not willing to accept what seems to me an extremely unfair arrangement. I deserve that money, and because I will not even consider giving it up, I have made a decision never to marry again. I would be thrilled to have another loving relationship and significant man in my life – but we would live together rather than marry this time. My father and husband are taking care of me now, and I'm going to make sure that never changes.

XXV

Throughout my life, I have had many surgeries. And I worry each time I'm in the hospital because I know from my own experience that you can go in one way and come out worse. Or, as in Neil's case, not come out at all. Unfortunately, sometimes there's just no choice in the matter.

Doctors inserted screws and a cable in my back because I have curvature of the spine. I've also had hip surgery, but I am still in pain. I need to change positions frequently when I am in my wheelchair because any weight on my hipbones and buttocks hurts, and my legs get numb.

When people with cerebral palsy are injured, it takes them longer to recover than someone who is in good health. And more than just the injured area will be sore. Each body part affects another one. For example, if I injure my wrist, my whole arm or my entire side could also hurt for quite awhile. My muscles tighten when I am in pain, and won't relax, causing the pain to increase and last a long time.

Because of the spasms of my muscles and tendons, extreme weather conditions bother me, too. I am in even greater pain when it becomes either very hot or very cold. And, if it is windy, I have difficulty breathing. The wind literally takes my breath away.

Cerebral palsy has taken both a physical and an emotional toll on me. As the years passed and my disorder progressed, I not only lost my mobility, but also my privacy. I could walk with help and braces on my legs until I was twelve years old, but my condition worsened after surgery. By the time I was twenty, I could no longer stand, and had to be lifted like a baby – from my wheelchair to the bed, or from the bed to the toilet. This is the time when a person with physical challenges must resign herself to a total loss of privacy. It is a time when you have to accept the fact that someone else will now have to be involved in every personal care issue of your life – whether it's bathing you, cleaning you after a bowel movement, or changing your sanitary napkins. It can't be helped, but believe me, it gets to you.

Others may think that this is something people with challenges get used to – particularly if they have been dealing with these issues all their lives. But you never get used to it and, in fact, it gets worse as you get older. It's much more embarrassing to be cleaned up after an accident when you are an adult than it is when you are a child.

Anyone who thinks this shouldn't bother a person has no idea how humiliating it feels. Personally, although I know I can't help it, I am still very hard on myself when I do have an accident. It makes me disappointed and sad. I have a specific image in my mind of what my adult self should look like. And being cleaned up like a baby does not fit that image.

Still, I try to keep an upbeat attitude as best I can. If I do have an accident, I don't let it spoil my entire day. I can't. That would accomplish nothing. I try not to make a big deal of the situation because that would also make the people around me feel uncomfortable. Sometimes, I may even laugh, but it's really nothing but nervous laughter. People may misinterpret my laughter, but I don't for one minute think it is comical - particularly when I know that wetting myself will probably mean spending the rest of the day in bed while my Hoyer sling is washed and dried. At times like these, I especially require a compassionate attendant. I don't need anyone belittling me when I am trying to cope with my own self-consciousness.

XXVI

The people who have been a part of my adult life have ranged from phenomenal to malicious. Some I will never forget for their kindness, and some for their cruelty. Many touched my heart, while others left permanent scars on it.

Not long ago, I was lucky enough to reconnect with a very special lady. Samantha was an essential part of my life many years ago. I met her when I was in my early 20s. She was a bus driver who transported me to the day program called The Place. Sam was a lot of fun, and used to take a group of us bowling quite regularly, and even camping once in awhile. She made me laugh and enjoy my life. Although we lost touch with each other about 20 years ago, I never forgot how important she was to me.

I was thrilled when I ran into Sam's daughter while I was out shopping recently. She told me how to reach her mother, and I was able to invite her to my housewarming party. I was so excited that she was able to make it! Sam loves elephants, and she gave me one as a housewarming gift. She wants me to think of her when I look at it. As much as I love and appreciate that elephant, I don't need something tangible to remind me of someone as unique and wonderful as Sam.

At the complete opposite end of the spectrum from Samantha was Doris who had a mental disability. She didn't start out as my personal care attendant. Initially, her boyfriend Andrew held that position. However, he was sent to jail, and since Doris was his backup, she took over in his place. At first, I thought things would be all right. After all, at times when I didn't have a phone or anyone to stay overnight with me, Doris would take me to her house to sleep.

However, when United Cerebral Palsy stopped mailing her paychecks on time, Doris got fed up and wouldn't come to work. She left me completely alone in my apartment for several days. When her 14 year old daughter and 13 year old niece came to check on me, they noticed that I was terribly uncomfortable and scratching my vaginal area. They called 911, and had me taken to the hospital. An internal examination uncovered the cause of my distress. I had fleas – both inside and out. It was quite obvious that I was not getting proper care. This was neglect of the worst kind!

Since Doris and my other attendants were not getting paid, I eventually lost all my workers, and Adult Protective Services moved me out of the apartment. It was then that Doris took me to her daughter's home to live. At the time, it seemed like a kindhearted thing for her to do, but I was soon to learn differently.

This was a full house even before I arrived. Doris, her two daughters, and eight grandchildren already lived there, with no child support coming in. I assumed that since I was moving in with a family, I would be safe. I didn't know yet that it was one extraordinarily dysfunctional family. Little did I suspect the heinous torment I would soon have to endure.

It wasn't long before I was being physically abused not only by Doris, but also by other members of her family. One of her daughters would stand on my feet, and threaten me by holding lit matches in my face. Her grandson actually cut my feet with a knife, and Doris herself devised numerous ways to inflict pain on me. She choked me and dug her fingernails into my neck. She slapped me and hit me with her fists, and withheld my food and drinks. She listened to my phone calls, and instructed me what to say and what not to say. If I accidentally urinated on my clothes, she cut them off of me. At times, she made me sleep on the kitchen floor, and if I urinated there, she would cancel my rides so I couldn't go out. Neither my family nor United Cerebral Palsy knew where I was, so I was literally Doris' prisoner for eight hellish months.

When Doris' boyfriend Andrew got out of jail, he and Doris moved me into their house with them. I didn't have a bed the first night we moved in. My brother Michael still had not returned my phone calls asking for one. So after Doris left to spend the night at her mother's Andrew put me on their mattress with him. Unfortunately, we overslept the next morning and when she came home and saw us together, she was seething with jealousy. Nothing inappropriate had happened between Andrew and me, but she was still furious. In retaliation, Doris, her daughter, and her niece dragged me up the stairs, scraping my back on the edge of every step along the way. If my brother had gotten me a bed, I would not have been on a mattress with Andrew. I would not have been dragged up the steps, and it's possible that my back would not be in the poor condition that it is today. I place partial blame for that on Michael.

A couple of the workers at Making Choices for Independent Living were becoming suspicious about what was going on in that house. It was obvious from my answers during our telephone conversations that something was not quite right. Since Doris was monitoring everything I said, I'm sure my tone of voice tipped them off. An MCIL housing specialist, James, came for a home visit, and didn't like what he saw. Doris was angry that he came, and exceedingly irritated that she had to bring me downstairs to meet with him.

Thank God, Andrew, his mother, and MCIL helped me plan an escape. If it weren't for them, I don't know what would have become of me. MCIL still owed Doris and her daughter money, and told them that if they wanted to get paid, I personally would have to come into the office and get their check. They knew it was the only way Doris would let me out of the house. Doris' daughter carried me outside to a cab, and sent me off to MCIL and freedom. As it turned out, they never did get paid, so they refused to return my suitcases and important papers that I had left at their house. I temporarily stayed with my old friend Odessa at her apartment, and later moved in with the Gibson family.

Somehow, Doris had to be taught a lesson. She had to learn that just because she was physically stronger than me, it did not give her the right to take advantage of that and abuse me. Consequently, I took her to court for mistreatment. The judge listened carefully as I recounted the horrors I endured at her hands. He convicted her, and told her that if it were up to him, he would sentence her to two life terms plus ten years in prison.

As unbelievable as it must have seemed to everyone, I actually wrote a letter asking the judge to show Doris leniency. My compassion was not directed particularly to her but more toward the rest of her family. There were eight children involved and they received no child support. I had seen them go days with nothing to eat. In fact, watching them without food made me more cognizant of wasting food myself, and angry with others who do. This was a family with enough problems already, and I knew that sending Doris to jail would negatively impact them all. I didn't want to be responsible for breaking up a family, no matter what they had done to me. I just wanted to make the point that she could not get away with abuse.

Although the judge would have preferred a much harsher sentence, because of my recommendation, he ordered Doris to receive behavioral counseling and to perform community service. She would also be on probation for six to eight years. I was satisfied with the outcome. My ordeal was over and Doris was punished – but I would never forget.

XXVII

Today's fears come from my past experiences. Although
many years have gone by, some of them are branded inside of me.
I will remember them all. It would be impossible not to. When I
reflect on what has happened to me, I am reminded that
unfortunately history could repeat itself. There are more people in
the world like Doris than anyone can imagine. I am aware that the
possibility of being hurt again today is great.

I tend to keep my emotions buried deep inside for a long
while – and I've come to realize that many people with cerebral
palsy or other challenges also find it difficult to put the past behind
them. My own feelings, especially negative ones, linger just below
the surface of my mind. Then they manifest themselves as
suspicions, and prevent me from becoming close to people when I
first meet them. As unfair as it is, it is hard for me to give
someone a chance to prove him or herself right away. It takes time
for people to earn my trust. They often misinterpret my feelings,
and think that I am blaming everyone in the world for my past bad
experiences. I'm not – I'm just fearful that there will be more.

Memories of abuse will last as long as I live. It is imperative
that my staff understand how the past affects the present. Even
now, I jump if someone taps me on the shoulder and I didn't see
them coming. This is a leftover fear caused by Doris who often
came up from behind without warning, and proceeded to hurt me.

The one positive aspect of all this fear and suspicion is that
they have made me a much less vulnerable person than before.
When I am working with a new person, I know the red flags to
watch for and I am a great deal more cautious now. Background
checks of all new hires are conducted thoroughly, and I speak with
people who have firsthand information about prospective

employees. I need to know exactly what kind of position I am putting myself into. I have to. My *own* background demands it.

XXVIII

Easy-going Jacquie is gone. There was a time when not much frazzled me, but when everyone I trusted let me down, it had a negative and permanent effect on me. What was intended to be a good move for me, resulted in an episode that would cause me an excessive amount of emotional distress.

My service coordinator suggested that an agency called Creative Options might be an appropriate residential choice for me. It was supposed to be a nice place to live where I would be cared for, and supplied with everything I needed to lead a comfortable life. People who lived there allegedly could come and go as they pleased.

It didn't take me long to realize that everything my service coordinator heard about Creative Options was a lie. What went on behind closed doors was a completely different scenario altogether. But, it took months for anyone to believe me.

I had to buy most of my own food, personal care items, and toiletries. Almost nothing was provided there. What food they did supply was awful. I wasn't given my medications, and I was denied enemas when I needed them. Consequently, I became very sick, and had to be hospitalized. Naturally, Creative Options covered up their neglect. Imagine trying to get help with your problems, and regardless of how many times you repeat yourself, no one hears or believes you. My frustration was beyond description.

As for people being able to leave and return to the facility at will, that wasn't true either. No one had that personal freedom. I couldn't even come home when I wanted to! I was the only person at Creative Options who wasn't allowed to have a key to our house. No matter where I was, what I was doing, or when I was finished, I had to wait for the rest of the residents to get in before I could go home. Quite often, I would have to bide my time at

United Cerebral Palsy's day program until after 4 o'clock just waiting to leave.

It was during those long hours that I became close friends with Tony. He worked for Yellow Transportation and had an office at United Cerebral Palsy. We would visit and chat to pass the time before my ride came to take me home. Tony began to notice that my trips to the day program were becoming rather sporadic. Sometimes, even though I had arranged for transportation, when the driver came to pick me up at Creative Options, he was told I was staying home, and was sent away. Tony started to wonder if something was wrong there. I explained to him what was happening, and he solved the problem for me. From then on, the driver would have to see me personally to confirm any changes in my plans.

In the eight months that I resided at Creative Options, I never received proper care. My anger was slowly building over time, but one incident finally pushed me over the edge. Some visitors came to see me and, although I was right in my room, they were told I was not home. This blatant lie was the last straw for me, and it called for immediate action on my part.

One day when it was time to leave United Cerebral Palsy's day program, and go back to Creative Options, I simply refused to get on the bus. I was determined not to spend another minute there! When it became obvious to everyone that I was stubborn enough not to budge, they called the police thinking I would listen to them. I became so distressed that the police said I should go to the hospital. They promised me if I calmed down, cooperated with them, and went along willingly to the hospital, they would take me to a hotel later.

Unfortunately, I was naïve enough to believe their lies. But, after I was discharged from the hospital, I was involuntarily admitted to a mental institution in Pennsylvania! I was stunned, and terribly hurt by this unbelievable deception! My faith in everyone disintegrated at this point. United Cerebral Palsy had actually assisted Creative Options and the police in this entrapment. These were people who should have been helping me, and now I could no longer trust them. Their betrayal was completely devastating.

I was totally isolated at the institution – trapped in a hopeless situation with no end in sight. My family never called or came to see me while I was there. I felt so alone. I was sick of everything. I was tired of fighting, and ready to give up. I didn't want to live anymore. The despair that I felt was so intense that I actually prayed to die in my sleep.

Finally, after eight lonely and frightening days, they were ready to send me back to Creative Options, but I said, "No!" I couldn't continue to live under those conditions. In the end, I was released to Mrs. Gibson and went home to stay with her once again.

Yes, easy-going Jacquie is gone for good, and the old Jacquie is not coming back. I have been let down too many times to remain the same person. People will have to accept me the way I am now. No one will walk over me again. The bitterness deep inside of me is fueled by a past that can't be changed.

XXIX

As my experience with Creative Options proves, selecting the right agency to support you is a critical decision. Be sure to visit agencies in person, but keep in mind that your initial impression can often be misleading. In fact, probably eight out of ten times, what you see during a scheduled visit will be totally different from reality. Naturally, you will need to meet with the administrators but their job is to convince you to come onboard with them. Therefore, they will make certain that everyone and everything presents an impeccable appearance.

A key strategy in the selection process is to interview people who are being supported by the agency. For complete honesty and an objective opinion, if possible interview them in another location. Try to arrange to meet with them in a place where they feel comfortable enough to speak freely and openly. It is the most ideal way to get an undistorted view of how things will be if you are with that agency and trying to advocate for yourself.

The most desirable agencies to me are those who have a mission statement that involves person centered planning. Those are the ones that won't try to fit you into a box or specific category, and that support people with all types of disabilities instead of just one. Person centered planning enables you to be in charge of your life and make most decisions on your own. Your plan is their plan and will be implemented as completely as possible. I feel it would be in your best interest to find an agency with that type of philosophy.

After many years, I transferred from my original agency to another more progressive one. I had been supported by United Cerebral Palsy for most of my life, and it was time to "roll on." Although United Cerebral Palsy paints a perfect image of itself on television and radio commercials, the reality is quite different. They profess to enable people to live independently, but their definition of independence is nothing like mine. To me, independent living means having my own individual apartment with the support staff that I need. Their idea of independent living is an apartment with three, four, or even five other people plus staff. This is an agency that doesn't look beyond a person's disability at the *whole* person, and sees only what you can't do. They believe that if you need a lot of physical assistance, then you are very vulnerable and can't possibly be on your own. They often seem to forget that a person can still have a very good mind. It is their belief that an assisted living situation is the best that you can do.

Somewhere along the way, United Cerebral Palsy as an agency has transferred its focus from the people they support to how much money they can make. There was a time when roommates who had similar abilities would share an apartment so they could interact well with each other. Now, people are clumped together based on how much money they have, or according to their parents' salaries. This results in many mismatched roommates, often pairing up someone who has severe mental retardation with another person who doesn't.

I became increasingly dissatisfied with my support at United Cerebral Palsy. Once I moved into my own apartment, I didn't require much assistance from them anymore. Even though I didn't ask for much, when I did, I rarely got what I needed. Sometimes, my requests were just passed around their office, and never addressed. The agency's mission should be person-oriented but, in my opinion, it no longer is. The organization has changed immensely over the years. Something is seriously wrong when a person *with* cerebral palsy, like me, wants out of an agency called United Cerebral Palsy. That just shouldn't be.

XXX

I switched to an agency called Shared Support, Inc. It was an exciting opportunity for me because of how self-directed this agency is. Individuals write up their own plan of care, and the agency supports their clients in the implementation of that plan. This is an innovative idea since most other agencies make a plan for you.

In addition, now that I am with Shared Support, I make the final decisions on hiring my own staff and establish guidelines for them. For most of my adult life, United Cerebral Palsy has handled my staff and there have been numerous problems that have come up. When they got someone who worked from their heart and truly cared about me, they overworked them. Sometimes, the good attendants had to pick up the slack from the lousy ones by fixing their mistakes or completing their unfinished work. The good and the bad workers were often paid the same wage. Eventually, the best ones got fed up with the situation and left.

Since I am completely in charge of my own staff now, I handle things much differently. My attendants get paid according to their output. If someone finishes their work, they get their full salary. If they don't finish, they get partial pay; and if someone finishes a task left incomplete from another attendant then that person gets extra wages. There is no money to waste. My new philosophy on salary is: "If you do half the work, you get half the pay."

Fortunately, I have had the guidance of some very helpful people in my life. In their own way, each has taught me a lesson regarding how to handle my staff. Antonio from United Cerebral Palsy reminded me that I am the boss, and to take charge. If my employee and I have agreed on a set schedule, but he or she decides to take time off with only one hour's notice – I have the right to tell them they can't. Antonio outlined the steps to take if staff members miss too much work. Give them two verbal warnings, followed by two written warnings if the behavior continues. The next step should be two weeks off without pay, and a report to their supervisor. Not showing up for work demonstrates a complete lack of respect for me. That's unacceptable, so after their two weeks off, I can decide whether or not to continue their employment. Antonio also believed that just one act of violence – even if it only involved breaking something in anger – was cause for immediate dismissal.

Tex, a person with his own challenges, had three personal care attendants. The method by which he paid them influenced me to model the same system today. It made perfect sense to me when he explained that his attendants were paid according to the amount of work they did. Linda, a care provider I hired through Tex, agreed with his idea concerning wages. I am still indebted to Antonio, Tex, and Linda for what I learned from each one of them.

I am also handling all of the paperwork for the hiring of my staff, and I'm responsible for their time sheets. In the past, workers mailed their timesheets directly to United Cerebral Palsy themselves. Since the changeover to Shared Support, it is solely up to me to make sure my staff is paid on time. I am completely capable of that task, and was willing and ready when I took on that new responsibility. The bottom line now is that I am the boss – a completely different setup than with United Cerebral Palsy. Shared Support, Inc. works for Jacqueline Speciner.

XXXI

A good service coordinator can be a tremendous asset and a strong advocate for you. He or she can secure additional services or medication for you – basically get you what you can't get for yourself. On the other hand, if a service coordinator becomes too powerful, that can work against you. Twice, I have had service coordinators take control away from me. They did what they thought was best for me, even though I disagreed. You must find someone who is forceful but not overbearing - one who will respect your wishes and opinions.

A service coordinator along with someone from your support agency, a psychologist, and perhaps family members can help you establish an Individual Program Plan, or IPP. This is a set of goals and objectives to be met within a specific timeframe that you write for yourself. They could range anywhere from learning to write your name to securing a job by a certain date. As indicated by its name, everyone's IPP will be applicable solely to that particular person according to what he or she wants to accomplish in life.

I am fortunate to have an additional means of support called a Circle of Friends. This is an innovative method which I highly recommend to everyone. An ideal Circle of Friends is made up of people who fill a variety of roles in your life, and who feel comfortable with you. They can be neighbors or friends who help you out. They can be people who work for you such as care attendants, or they can be relatives. The choices are completely up to you. You extend the invitations to join, and let each person know what you need from them. You also determine how often you'd like to meet with the group. Some members will attend every meeting, while others might pick and choose depending on the reason for getting together. The Circle and its members fluctuate as everyone's functions and your needs change.

Those attending a typical Circle meeting of mine might include my service coordinator, my support broker, an employee or two, plus a number of advocates and friends. Generally, we discuss any concerns or problems that I have at the time, such as how to terminate an undesirable employee. They can *suggest* possible solutions for me to consider. I make the decision whether to take their advice or not. We may then move on to talk about my desires and plans for the future. If anyone has been working on a special project for me, then he or she will update me with a report. Occasionally, my finances will be a topic of discussion. In the past, we have talked at length about what my yearly budget includes.

XXXII

Naturally, everyone's budget is different, tailored to their own individual needs. My latest budget pays for a nursing service to check on my health and well-being every three months, a lifeline emergency response system, and some adaptive equipment that I need. It covers rehabilitation after surgery in my own home, rather than in a nursing facility. In addition, it pays the complete cost of two ADAPT conferences per year.

To assist me in my plan to become gainfully employed, this budget will also pay for a job coach and wireless Internet service. My hope is to secure a grant which would enable me to purchase part of a van business. I would actually like to receive training to learn how to run a company, so I can become a partner. With the proper supports and adaptations, I could also hold a secretarial position. It's possible that I can get funding from the Department of Vocational Rehabilitation in order to attain this goal.

Being a partner in a van business would be beneficial to me in a number of ways. First of all, I would be employed which is very important to me, plus I think it would be an interesting job. Especially appealing though, is the fact that it would afford me the opportunity to have my own van. My life would change immensely for the better if that happened. It is one of my greatest desires – to own a van and hire two drivers. I know it would entail a lot of paperwork. It would mean getting insurance for the van, the drivers, and me – plus a special license for the drivers. Whatever the process though, it would be worth it to gain more independence and greater freedom.

There is also money in my budget to hire a fiscal management service, which I have done. Choosing such a service is, of course, another very personal decision. As with any other service, you need to research your options thoroughly, and compare and contrast companies. That is the only way you can make an informed selection. I had two services to consider – MedSource Community Services and The Arc of Anne Arundel County. After reviewing packets of information from both, I decided that MedSource Community Services was the better choice for me – based on what it had to offer in conjunction with my particular needs.

All of my Developmental Disability Administration (DDA) funds are now in the hands of MedSource to be disbursed according to my wishes. It pays each person who works for me. However, I authorize who gets paid and how much they get, as specified in my Individual Plan. If I decide to make a change, I must send a letter to DDA along with a copy of my entire, current budget for them to review. They have the option of approving or denying my request for a change.

Among other things, MedSource prints and mails paychecks to my employees in a *timely* fashion. They review disbursement requests to verify that they comply with my budget. They also print and distribute individual financial statements and 1099 forms. They keep general ledger accounts and client files for me. In addition, I received 3.5 hours of phone contact in the first three months of service, plus I have 30 minutes of phone consultation each month thereafter.

MedSource considers itself a "business consultant." They do not make decisions on how my money is spent. That is still my prerogative. They give opinions and make recommendations, but it is my choice whether or not to follow them. There is no penalty if I turn down their advice. They still support me regardless of my decisions. MedSource states that its "role is to listen, educate, and provide technical support when requested." The service does not impose its views on anyone and realizes that it must be "flexible and innovative" to meet the needs of its clients.

MedSource assists me with my financial and personnel management. It is a satisfactory and cost-effective service well worth the initial enrollment fee and monthly charges. I strongly suggest that you retain a fiscal management service to help guide you through the maze of your monetary paperwork.

XXXIII

There are numerous tools available to help people with disabilities live as independently as possible. In order to be self-reliant, and have all of your needs met, utilize as many resources as you can. Although you may find means of assistance at the library, in newspapers and phone books, or on the Internet, pay close attention to any recommendations received by word of mouth. Anyone who can say, "Been there, done that" usually has accurate information to share. Information you can trust.

The Maryland Department of Transportation has mobility vans accessible for people with special needs. Each prospective rider must submit an application, and proof from a physician that they qualify for the service. If your application is approved, it is good for three years. After that, you must reapply.

My advice from personal experience is that if you have any other means of transportation, use it. Although I am very glad that I have access to this service, it has a number of aggravating glitches. The vans are notoriously late, and may leave you waiting somewhere for hours. The MTA schedules do not always coincide to the times that you need a ride. You may have to be picked up much earlier than necessary for your appointment, just to fit into MTA's timeframe. It's also impossible for you to go anywhere at the last minute. To arrange a ride, you are required to call by 5:00 p.m. the night before. If you forget, you are out of luck. There's no flexibility, and MTA is most definitely "in the driver's seat."

They really should, at the very least, have an "in a bind" transportation plan available. This could be utilized for an occasion that's not an emergency and does not demand an ambulance, but requires you to get somewhere without much notice. And you could arrange a ride for that same day. Maybe a friend calls and wants you to go shopping, or maybe you just found out that a relative is sick and you want to visit him. Right now, there is no leeway for such situations, and there should be. If you absolutely have no other options, then it is worth tolerating the inconveniences of MTA. Without a doubt, it's preferable to staying home.

XXXIV

One glance at my calendar and it's apparent that I am living my life as positively as I can. Life is definitely a challenge, but I can choose to stay active or stare at the four walls. My choice is to utilize the skills that I have, so I don't lose them. I'm not afraid to take chances. If I were, my life would be stagnant. It's never beneficial to be idle, so I do everything I can to keep myself busy and productive.

When I was in my mid-twenties, I participated as a volunteer in an after-school program. It was a school for troubled teens, and I hope I made an impression on them. My goal was to help them realize what their lives would be like if they ended up in a wheelchair. At the time, they had no physical reason to need one, but if they continued following their self-destructive paths and ended up shot that could quickly change.

I went to their school twice a week for seven months, and although some of the students had smart mouths, on the whole they were respectful to me and interested in what I had to say. They were shocked at some of my experiences, and astonished when they saw my wedding video. I suppose they didn't expect that someone in my condition would ever get married. I never want to project a completely negative perspective on my life. I wanted them to know that – yes – they *could* live their life in a wheelchair like me, but it would be complicated. Based on their firsthand observations of my challenges, I hope that at least some of them changed their circumstances, and chose a less dangerous way of life.

Later, a similar position became available that paid a small stipend. Although I enjoyed my volunteer work, I certainly had no objection to receiving some money for my time. This job entailed going to a number of different schools, and speaking to children of various age levels. I talked to them about my childhood and my relationship with my parents. I explained about my many physical needs, including the help I require in the bathroom. I covered both the positive and negative aspects of my life, as well as my personal accomplishments. It's important for children to have the opportunity to satisfy their curiosity, so I always included a question and answer session. I made certain that my explanations were age appropriate and on a level that each child could clearly understand. To a four year old, I would equate the wheels of my wheelchair to my legs. Yet to an eighteen year old, I would explain in detail the muscular problems caused by cerebral palsy.

One job that gives me great satisfaction today is participating in training conferences. On a few occasions, I have been compensated by Shared Support, Inc. to instruct people in formulating Individual Program Plans using the person-centered planning format. I find this work quite gratifying, and expect to do more of it in the future.

My life is, without a doubt, a full one – brimming with social engagements, too. I regularly attend The Lord's Church, and receive great comfort from its leader Bishop Elliott. I go on outings with the singles' ministry and enjoy the camaraderie of the other participants. I love to go shopping, and particularly out to eat.

My most meaningful activity however, is definitely my involvement in ADAPT, a disability rights organization. It is devoted to freeing people from nursing homes and changing our country's long-term care system. It has staged national protests in fourteen different cities across the country – from Las Vegas to Baltimore, from Orlando to Seattle, and many locations in between. I personally have participated in ADAPT protests in San Francisco and Washington, DC, joining others in exercising our First Amendment rights. It is a grassroots organization, and we fight for people who physically can't fight for themselves, or for people who want change but are not comfortable personally using direct action. I am very passionate about joining my voice to the emphatic cry of this powerful organization.

XXXV

I do have a wish though that would make my life even more complete. If I could rub a magic lamp and have a dream come true, people may be surprised by what I'd ask for. Would I love to be able to run downstairs, out the door, jump in my car, and drive away? Of course I would, but that would not be my wish. Would I want to be completely self-sufficient and not need anyone to take care of me? Yes, I would... but I still have a greater desire than that.

For my entire adult life, I have yearned to be someone's mother. I adore children, and would have loved the opportunity to be pregnant. People with cerebral palsy are capable of having a normal pregnancy, but that chance was stolen from me when I had a hysterectomy. My physical condition would have made pregnancy a painful ordeal for me – but I would have suffered the discomfort gladly and without complaint. I regret missing the wondrous miracle of carrying a child beneath my heart.

Children mean a great deal to me, and Neil wanted children, too. So, when we were married, we inquired about adoption. Naturally, we realized that we could not manage an infant on our own. We knew we could do very little to care for a baby, and would have needed a great deal of extra help. So, we looked into adopting a child between the ages of six and eight years old. However, each time we called an adoption agency, we were met with rude and negative responses. Once they knew the extent of care that Neil and I needed, everyone decided it wouldn't be fair to a child to be placed with us. They were even crass enough to suggest that we were mainly interested in the money we would receive for a child's start-up care. Being rejected as adoptive parents was a major disappointment to both of us.

Despite the opinions of the adoption agencies, I believe in my heart that I could have been a good mother. I have learned a great deal by watching other people with their children. Even the way I was brought up would have influenced how I would raise my own child. My upbringing mostly taught me what mistakes not to make. My treatment of children would be vastly different from what took place in my family.

Although they didn't always treat me with respect, my parents did teach me to respect others. It's one of the few things they did right. This is an important trait that I would pass on to my own children. The valuable lesson of The Golden Rule will never go out of style.

Without a doubt, I wouldn't make one child take full responsibility for another one. Of course, I would expect them to watch out for each other – as all family members should. However, I saw firsthand how my sisters resented having to take care of me, and how they rebelled. Children are entitled to enjoy their childhood. They shouldn't have to perform an adult's tasks, day after day. It is one of the reasons my sisters ran away from home. They got fed up doing my mother's job for her.

I would treat each child as an individual according to his or her personality and age. Bedtimes would be set, but would vary by age. My siblings went to bed whenever they felt like it. I prefer more structure than that.

My children would also have chores to earn money for clothes. That's how they start learning financial responsibility, and it teaches them that everything in life will not be handed to them. It would have been good for me to have helped around the house when I was young. It would have been useful preparation for the time when I was expected to pitch in and help care for my own place.

In addition, I would show love for my children by being deeply involved in their lives. I'd be more than a bystander. I'd be front and center at all of their games, at their shows, and anything else they participated in. I would be their most fervent cheerleader. And I would be there, not out of a sense of duty, but to demonstrate to them that they mean the world to me.

But most importantly, I would never, ever hit a child. There are many other ways to handle stress, and much better options for discipline. My child would have a time-out, or I would withhold privileges. Hitting does nothing to solve a problem, and instead creates another one. It teaches children that violence is an acceptable solution to a confrontation. It sends a completely wrong message. One my child would never learn from me.

I know I could have raised a child the right way – if only I had been given the chance. Because I was denied that miraculous privilege, I am especially angry when I see others prove they don't deserve to be parents. My message to them is this… Children should not be made to pay for your anger. They are not to blame, so please don't take it out on them. They didn't ask to be born. One way or another that was your decision. You laid down; you made love, and chose to have a baby. Or you had eggs implanted in order to conceive. Maybe you even adopted. Whatever the method, your children had no say in the matter. They are true blessings, and that's how they should be treated. I just wish I could have been blessed with one myself.

XXXVI

My family... What can I say about my own family? Our relationship is as complicated as nuclear physics, yet as simple as taking a breath. Despite their intolerance, despite their indifference, and despite the numerous times they have disappointed me – together they comprise a patchwork quilt that I desperately want to wrap around myself. The simple truth is that I love them.

When I moved out on my own, it was to gain a modicum of independence. It was never my intention to leave my family behind, or eliminate them from my life. Yet, as years go by, I see them less and less. This is their choice, most definitely not mine.

I have tried to reestablish a relationship with my family, but without success. One of my sisters visits occasionally, but I only see my mother about twice a year. I'd give anything to be closer to my mom, and I feel a physical ache inside knowing that's unlikely to happen. My efforts to contact her are often ignored. She hardly ever responds to messages that I leave. There is usually no acknowledgement that I even called.

It has been 26 years since I moved out of my mother's house. Things definitely haven't always gone smoothly. I know I've made some mistakes, but I've never given up striving to be as self-sufficient as possible. In spite of some unbearable circumstances, I have never gone running back home – not even once. I'm proud of myself for that, and my mother should be, too.

The emotional anguish becomes even more intense whenever there is a holiday. I want to be with my family, but they never invite me to join them. It is so depressing to know that my entire family is together for a holiday or other special event, and I am excluded. I am an outsider to them.

When I specifically asked if I could visit one Christmas, I was told "no." I tried to convince my mother that I wouldn't be any trouble. No one would have to transport me. No one would have to feed me, or take me to the bathroom. They wouldn't have to care for me in any way. I would pay for my own transportation, and pay my attendant to come with me. Instead of being reassured by my arrangements, my mother said that would cost me too much money. I told her I really didn't care about the money, that I just wanted to be with everyone. Her reply was that she would visit me sometime after Christmas and we would go to the mall. There was simply no changing her mind. And she never did come that year.

I wish I knew the real reason that my family literally bans me from all of their celebrations. I suspect that they are afraid I will have an embarrassing accident while I am in their house. Whatever the explanation, how can they be so oblivious to the pain they are causing me?

On the very rare occasions that my mother and stepfather do come to see me, I have to erect an imaginary shield to protect myself from the wretched memories of my childhood. I cannot force myself to call Earl "dad" like my mother wants me to. He mistreated her and me, so I will never be able to refer to him using that affectionate term. It is difficult enough to cope with the fact that he and my mother are still together. Although I love her a lot, her lack of self-respect by allowing him to remain in her life makes it impossible for me to respect her.

Earl does treat me better than he did when I was a child but I still think if he were antagonized enough, he would mistreat me again. Because of his abusive personality, I can't believe that after he retired from the post office, he got a job at a school for children with disabilities! It frightens me that to this day, he is still working there. Personally, I will be terrified of him until he dies, and I absolutely believe that I would not have lived if I had stayed at home. He might have easily killed me, and convinced everyone that it was an accident. How could I ever possibly call him "dad?"

Because I see my mother so infrequently, I am afraid that the same thing will happen with her as it did with my father. She has already had by-pass surgery, and she shows the beginnings of

Alzheimer's disease. I worry because I am not really certain how serious my mother's condition is right now. No one is keeping me informed, and I'm terrified that one day I will get a call telling me that she died. I can't bear the thought of going through that again.

I've always considered it a blessing that I moved out of her house before she became sick. Her health problems coupled with my physical challenges would have been overwhelming for her. Whenever my mother does visit, I hate for her to leave because I never know when, or if, I'll get to see her again.

Obviously, a close relationship with my family is important only to me. Even my siblings don't seem interested in maintaining contact. As a result, I'm also completely uninvolved in my nieces' and nephews' lives. It upsets me terribly that I don't see them and hardly know anything about them.

Late last year, I was in the mall when a young woman approached me, and addressed me by name. She was my sister's daughter Courtney, and I didn't even recognize her. When I did realize who she was, I started to cry because I had not seen her since she was a teenager. I have no idea what my nieces and nephews are doing, and it leaves a huge void in my life. Courtney knew I had not seen her mother for years, and promised to give her my phone number. To date, however, I still have not received a call from my sister Jodell. As she said good-bye that day, Courtney hugged and kissed me, and told me she loved me. Running into Courtney was a pleasant surprise, but also an unhappy reminder of what I am missing.

And so, I must live my own life. My family is going on with their lives, so I must move on, too. I can't force them to be with me. I make my own family from the loving friends who surround me day after day. In fact, on the last two New Year's Eves, I made sure I was out with many of them. In 2004, I went to church and prayed. I enjoyed listening to the choir. However, the following year, I went to a masquerade party with all the trimmings. The dress was formal attire. Lots of my friends were there, and we had a champagne toast at midnight.

Gone are the times I had to make myself scarce on holidays, because the owners of the house where I lived wanted to entertain *their* family. I have my own apartment now, so I can go out or stay home and invite as many people over as I want. Maybe someday, when I invite my family to spend a holiday with me, they'll surprise me, and accept. Maybe… just maybe.

XXXVII

I have changed residences many times, and it seems that I've left each place on a negative note. Sometimes, my lack of patience caused me to lose my temper and get into an argument. Other times, there were financial complications. It seemed like there was always a reason for me to move on. It has taken many years, plenty of disappointments, and the unwavering determination of my support broker Gail, for me to reach the place where I am today. Gail helped turn a lifelong dream of mine into a wondrous reality – living in my very own apartment.

My present location is perfect. I have a variety of choices for shopping and many restaurants within "rolling" distance. That makes it possible for me to do those things on the spur of the moment.

I love going to the nearby mall, and enjoy getting out and about. I never mind interacting with people there, if they choose to approach me. I particularly love seeing children, and I don't mind talking about my condition with them. That's why when I am in public, I wish parents would not snatch their children away from me if they are inquisitive. This happens quite frequently, and it bothers me immensely when children are discouraged from asking questions. I don't consider their questions rude at all. Children should learn that cerebral palsy is not contagious, and they should be allowed positive interaction with people who have physical challenges. Yanking a child away from me, not only hurts me, but makes me sad for the child. Adults display their ignorance when they act like that, and at the same time, are passing their own prejudices on to their offspring. Let the child speak to me. I want them to ask me questions. I don't want them to be afraid of me because of my differences.

Unlike children who express bold curiosity, when I encounter adults they display varied reactions to me. Reactions can be from one end of the spectrum to the other. When I am shopping, store employees will either smother me with attention and help, or completely ignore me. Quite frankly, I don't care for either extreme. I like a little extra attention and some fussing over, but I don't want to be treated like a princess on a throne. Conversely, I don't want to feel like I am invisible either. Most probably, when adults don't know how to react to me, they choose not to react at all – and just pretend I'm not there.

There are even a few places where I hate to go alone, because of the contact I must have with the adults there. At the top of the list is the local courthouse. It seems to be staffed with the most insensitive adults on earth. If my paperwork isn't totally completed, they become impatient and don't want to take the time to help me. Even if my papers *are* in order, they dislike having to retrieve them from my tote bag. They make it obvious that they consider it a real inconvenience. It's a much more pleasant and stress free visit to the courthouse if someone can come with me to help. Although it's worth it to escape the rude treatment I often receive, it's not always possible to have another person along. Besides, I should be treated with dignity, and not made to feel like a burden to the courthouse employees. Children are so much less complicated to deal with.

An additional benefit of having my own apartment is that I can make plans when I want to, instead of having to work around another roommate's schedule. And no one can tell me to be quiet in my own home either. It is an entirely different world for me, and the freedom this affords me is powerful. I plan to stay here for awhile because it's a nice, convenient place. Eventually though, I want to get a bigger apartment with room for a home office for myself.

It is difficult, however, to plan meals for one person. That's one downfall of living by myself. I do everything I can to avoid wasting food. Sometimes, it's more efficient to eat out than to have a lot of leftovers from home-cooked meals. Often, I'll share what I have with friends or neighbors so I won't have to throw anything away. This one concern, however, is far outweighed by the liberating benefits of living alone.

It is a wonderful experience to be in my very own apartment. Someone else might take that for granted, but for me – not living in another person's house or sharing space with a roommate – is a unique pleasure and personal triumph for me.

XXXVIII

As I come to the end of my writing, I am at a peaceful place in my life. I am as self-sufficient as I can be, and I feel fulfilled. Finally, at age 48, my dreams are coming true.

My personal care attendant Nicole treats me with respect, and never raises her voice to me. Nothing I ask of her is too much trouble. She does exactly what I want – the way I want it done. If she does happen to have a different idea, she presents it to me in an appropriate manner. Nicole's not only dependable, she goes beyond her responsibilities. Her personal goal is to make me happy, and nothing upsets her more than if I am depressed. She loves working with me, and she actually says she hates to leave at the end of the day.

Although Nicole is only 26, she displays maturity greater than her years. She carries much weight on her young shoulders. Besides raising two small children, she often cares for her mother and her grandmother. And if someone else needs her, she finds a way to help them, too. For awhile she was also working two jobs and going to college. She recently graduated, and is truly an inspiration to me.

We have such a special relationship that she calls me her second mother. I try to help guide her on the right path as much as I can. She may not always like my suggestions, but she will listen to me without getting angry – and respects my opinions.

Yes, my life is good right now. I am active and happy. I am well-cared for – and I am surrounded by a circle of loving friends.

XXXIX

If you have a physical challenge and want to live on your own, you must have the will to make it work. Besides a strong desire for your own personal space, you need to remember that you are an adult and not allow yourself to be intimidated. There are a myriad of details to consider when choosing a place to live and the people to support you, but in the end it will be well worth it.

Remember that your personal needs and interests are of the utmost significance. Whether you are checking out the structure of an apartment or interviewing a potential caregiver, make sure they meet requirements set by you, and you alone.

There is no cookie cutter pattern to be used for everyone. Each person, even those with the same challenges, has specific, individual needs. Those needs may be determined by your level of physical ability or, just as importantly, by your own personal preferences.

And so... I leave you with this message:

If you know in your heart what you want, don't let *anyone* tell you *no*!!! You *can* do it! People will try to discourage you – but don't let them. Stand up for yourself and don't back down. I am living proof that with the right support, planning, and prayer, you can achieve your goals. Create a vision for yourself, and do everything in your power to secure the help you need so that your vision can become your reality.

I have persevered, and because of my perseverance have reached heights that no one else thought possible.

It has been a long journey with roadblocks along the way too numerous to count. But each hardship for me was also a learning experience – and from every pitfall, I have emerged stronger and better prepared to deal with my challenges! My hope for you is the same...

Afterword
By Phyllis Godwin

When I sat down for my job interview with Jacqueline Speciner, I had no idea what to expect. All I knew was that she was a 47 year old woman with cerebral palsy who wanted to write a book. She needed someone to help her, and I was applying for the position. I didn't realize that I was about to embark on an amazing journey through the life of this remarkable woman.

Jacquie had very specific ideas about what she wanted to say in her book. The very first thing she made clear to me was that she considers cerebral palsy a "challenge" instead of a "disability" – and I was not to use that word. I tried to come up with various ways to say "challenge" to keep from sounding too repetitious. It was very difficult and I finally got her permission to slip "disability" in on a few, very rare occasions. Jacquie prefers challenge because it is a more positive word – and despite all she has been through, her positive attitude is quite apparent.

Jacquie's goal in writing this book was twofold. It was to be a memoir but also a resource book for other people with physical challenges. She wanted to tell the story of her life, but also help people avoid some of the obstacles that she has experienced.

And so, in October 2005, Jacquie started talking to me while I listened and took notes. For seven months, I heard the ups and downs of her life – from birth through adulthood. There were times when I felt very sad for Jacquie and sickened by the way she had been treated. Other days I left thinking about how much she had overcome to get to where she is today. On more than one occasion, I told myself I would never complain about anything in my own life again. But most amazing is that Jacquie does not want anyone feeling sorry for her, and spends much of her time concerned about others.

During our months together, I got to know Jacquie quite well. She is a very compassionate person, and in her unselfish way, she began worrying about *my* family and friends. I felt she had more than enough worries of her own, but found that she always tries to look out for other people and offers ideas if they need help. Her thoughtfulness touched me.

I thoroughly enjoyed my time spent with Jacquie, and I am inspired by her perseverance to reach goals that so many people thought impossible for her. My job is over, but I will continue to keep in touch with Jacquie, and look forward to seeing her realize even more of her dreams!